End of Life Care

A Guide for Therapists, Artists and Arts Therapists

NIGEL HARTLEY

Foreword by Professor Dame Barbara Monroe

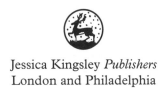

Jessica Kingsley *Publishers*
London and Philadelphia

First published in 2014
by Jessica Kingsley Publishers
73 Collier Street
London N1 9BE, UK
and
400 Market Street, Suite 400
Philadelphia, PA 19106, USA

www.jkp.com

Copyright © Nigel Hartley 2014
Foreword copyright © Barbara Monroe 2014
Cover artwork copyright © MAP Foundation

Library of Congress Cataloging in Publication Data
Hartley, Nigel.
  End of life care : a guide for therapists, artists and arts therapists / Nigel Hartley.
    pages cm
  Includes bibliographical references and index.
  ISBN 978-1-84905-133-0 (alk. paper)
  1. Terminal care. 2. Palliative treatment. 3. Art therapy. I. Title.
  R726.8.H367 2013
  616.02'9--dc23
                             2013024549

British Library Cataloguing in Publication Data
A CIP catalogue record for this book is available from the British Library

ISBN 978 1 84905 133 0
eISBN 978 0 85700 336 2

Printed and bound in Great Britain by Bell and Bain Ltd, Glasgow

For Mum and for Tom

Contents

Foreword

Individuals coming to the end of their lives often find themselves seeking ways to make sense of their current experiences, to set them in some sort of context and to understand and express their life story and its significance. Being able to tell our story, being listened to and heard, is a basic human need. Words are important tools in this task but not everyone, on every occasion, uses them with ease. The creative arts offer a wider variety of opportunities for self-exploration and expression. It has always seemed to me that one of the tragic consequences of our often death denying culture is that just when people most need social support, the world often retreats from them in embarrassment, anxiety and dismay, creating a kind of social death long before physical demise occurs. For many the creative arts can also provide a mechanism for exploration and expression in the company of others, sharing some aspects of experience but also hearing differences which deliver new insights for all involved. It is very depleting of the spirit to be always on the receiving end of care. It can confirm a passive patient status, that the individual is now someone to whom things are done, the object of professional ministrations and prescriptions. Care that heals, in addition to meticulous attention to physical needs, is care that creates partnerships, a temporary shared platform for mutual endeavour between therapists and patients and between patients and families and friends. As one dying individual put it to me: 'We are all up the same creek without a paddle.'

This important book describes practical ways for therapists, artists and arts therapists to set about delivering an effective professional offering in a wide variety of end of life care settings; ranging from outpatient services, inpatient units, the community and care homes and across all illnesses including dementia. The book is a pragmatic, realistic and forthright guide to the difficulties and rewards of being a rather unusual, sometimes isolated, often poorly understood professional; a sort of mythical tiger burning bright in the sometimes impenetrable forest of the efficient demands of medical and nursing structures. I have often teased Nigel Hartley and his talented team about their capacity to 'sprinkle fairy dust'. This is not a belittling comment. The walls of St Christopher's are vibrant with ever changing artwork. Visitors, patients and professionals all pause and take stock at these reflections of a life being lived, but coming to an end. I am so glad they are there – they are at the heart of what we do and demonstrate the value of those important relationship based spaces where the unexpected can happen. Most recently, amongst a set of powerful self-portraits, were hung a series of identical handkerchiefs decorated with very different images and messages. *'I am terminal but not extinct yet.' 'My heart is breaking, but I live on through my family and friends.' 'If I had to choose between loving and breathing, I would use my last breath to tell you I love you. Blow me a kiss.'*

The creative arts can cut through our painful defences to establish a dialogue in what was isolating silence. The description of the schools' programme in this book also shows us the power of the arts to help the development of emotional literacy about death, dying and bereavement. Society needs greater public engagement and confidence in these areas so that we can support one another as each one of us in turn faces the inevitability of the deaths of those close to us and ultimately our own. What I particularly admire about this book is its determination to be relevant. The current context of end of life care is clearly described with its resource constraints and necessary demands for cost effectiveness and the demonstration of value. It challenges professionals in the arts fields to focus on helping others to understand clearly and simply what it is that they do and why it might be of benefit and to pay attention to modifying approaches according to the very different settings in which care is delivered. It argues for an absolute but flexible focus on the individual patient, however brief the intervention, rather than a rigid professional insistence on a pre-determined therapeutic structure. Funding, supervision, recording, evaluation, education, research and many other issues are discussed. This attention to practical detail in such a text is unusual and welcome.

This is a brave book and now, more than ever, all practitioners in the field of end of life care need to initiate courageous conversations if we are to meet the ever growing need.

Professor Dame Barbara Monroe
Chief Executive
St Christopher's Group

Acknowledgements

I am indebted to those artists and therapists who have added their experiences, stories and expertise to the central chapters of this book, and also to all the patients, staff and volunteers who have contributed with either their personal stories which are included, or who over the years have inspired and motivated the ideas that are presented throughout. Personal thanks go to those who have funded many of the new projects discussed within the book, for example, Colin Russell, his fellow trustees and the benefactors of The Alfred and Peggy Harvey Trust, as well as the Arts Council, England. Thanks also go to Dame Barbara Monroe, the Senior Management Team and the Trustees of the St Christopher's Group, London, for continuing to support the growth and development of this work.

PART 1

History, Policy and Current Challenges

Chapter 1

Introduction

Why this book now?

The intention of this book is to give a clear and practical guide to what is required to work in, and what it is like to work as part of, the changing landscape of end of life care. As the majority workforces in most health care settings are nursing and medicine, the book aims to offer direction to a number of those professions which for whatever reason are occasionally marginalised, misunderstood and neglected, namely artists, therapists and arts therapists.

It is almost 25 years since I began working in end of life care, initially as a music therapist at London Lighthouse, a centre supporting those who were living with HIV/AIDS. Some years later I moved on to work at Sir Michael Sobell House, a large hospice in Oxford which is part of the Oxford Radcliffe Hospitals NHS Trust. I moved to St Christopher's in 2004, where I work as a senior manager responsible for overseeing most clinical activities across the organisation other than nursing and medicine. Although a team of artists is only one of a number of services I am now responsible for, I remain wholly committed to the usefulness of both the arts and other therapies within different health and social care settings, particularly those focussing on end of life care. This book is hopefully a testament to that commitment.

Alongside my early work in end of life care, I also worked in child, adolescent and adult mental health and with those living with physical and mental disability. I have also taught the arts in health and the arts therapies extensively both in the UK and in a range of other countries. In the late 1990s, I sat on the boards and chaired both the Association of Professional Music Therapists (UK) and also the British Society for Music Therapy, becoming the only person to chair both organisations simultaneously. This in turn led to a merger of both organisations and to the formation of the British Association of Music Therapy some years later.

One aim of this book is to share some personal experiences and thoughts, and in doing so to guide and motivate both artists and therapists who either currently work in end of life care, or who will work in the end of life care arena of the future, whatever that may look like. Stepping into a new job within an organisation which provides services to people during a particularly vulnerable time in their lives can often feel overwhelming and bewildering. For those people who are interested in working in end of life care or who find themselves working in the field with little preparation, it is hoped that this book will act both as a map and as a guide, demythologising and helping the process to be more simple and the services which are provided to be more straightforward and down to earth. It is certainly not an aim of this book to tell people 'how to do it' as my experiences have undoubtedly shown me that there are many different ways to provide successful services to individuals coming to the end of their lives. However, there is an intention to flag up some possible common misconceptions about working in this area, to urge a flexible and creative approach, and to dispel a few myths. It is also intended to demonstrate and persuade that many of the challenges and difficulties that you will face are universal and commonly shared with other practitioners, and that they can be met and overcome by sharing openly and honestly in order to try and not make the same mistakes repeatedly.

A major reason for writing this book at this moment in time is the significance and rapidity of the growth of current global economic and humanitarian challenges facing, and changes within, the health and social care sector. At present, we are experiencing a significant sense of turmoil, and any service provision requires a newly defined clarity and unambiguous rationale as well as needing to prove itself as being cost effective and relevant while consistently undergoing clinical self-scrutiny. Changes of such proportion are not straightforward at any time, but we must remember that with such transformation also comes possibility and potential. There has never been a more crucial time for health and social care professional groups and service providers to undertake some serious reflection and to explore the need to re-evaluate and reform themselves. This is true of all professional disciplines, but if some of the less mainstream occupations are unable to inspect and transform themselves at this time in order to become more useful, more relevant and more cost effective as part of a newly emerging future health and social care landscape, they could very well find themselves lacking, growing more irrelevant and potentially becoming side-lined and overlooked.

How is the book structured?

The book is divided up into three main sections:

1. History, policy and current challenges

2. Teamwork, communication and working in different contexts

3. Starting out, looking after yourself, research and development.

The final chapter concludes the book and reflects on some of the key themes while offering a resume of 'handy hints and tips'. Although the book is structured by presenting a number of chapters covering a range of important areas to be considered when working in end of life care, each chapter begins with a simple, helpful list of areas which are addressed within it. This is intended to give the reader the potential to dip in and out of the book when wanting to look quickly at certain key issues and information.

The first major section of the book contains three chapters which are written by me and cover matters such as the philosophy and history of the hospice movement, as well as focussing on key areas including strategic issues, current challenges and changes in the field. The second and third sections of the book contain useful input from current end of life arts and therapy practitioners.

Each of these chapters has an introduction and a concluding reflection from me focussing on some of the principal issues raised. The main body of each chapter is made up of material taken from the thoughts and work of a group of practitioners who work at St Christopher's, who share their encounters and their understanding from a range of different perspectives. I furnished each contributor with a list of headings, questions and ideas and asked them to respond to them from their own perspective and experiences. I then restructured their contribution to fit into an overall collective style.

Each person offers fresh, contemporary and up-to-date information on specific key areas which is relevant to both the experienced practitioner and also to the novice end of life care artist or therapist.

Although the book is targeted towards artists, therapists and arts therapists, it is of course intended that much of the information will be of use to other professional individuals coming from a range of differing disciplines and traditions.

The second major section of the book begins with Chapter 4 and introduces us to Tamsin Dives, who offers her experiences around working as part of a multi-disciplinary team, which is followed in the next chapter by Andy Ridley who shares his stories and knowledge of working with patients and families on a large inpatient unit.

Chapters 6 and 7 follow in a similar vein where we meet Mick Sands and Gerry Prince who tell us about working with day and outpatients and working in a variety of community settings. The latter offers some clear, practical advice when travelling around the community and working with patients and families in a range of different home contexts. This part of the book concludes with Gini Lawson, who takes us through a number of key issues which need consideration when supporting people through bereavement and loss.

The final section of the book begins by introducing us to Roberto Marcelo Sánchez-Camus in Chapter 9. Roberto shares his experiences of preparing for and being interviewed for a community artist position, as well as planning, preparing and carrying out projects with groups of people within a range of settings. Chapter 10 highlights the importance of supporting ourselves as we carry out our work in end of life care. These insights and experiences are proffered by Marion Tasker who has worked in this area for a number of years. Giorgos Tsiris, a recently qualified music therapist, takes us in a direct and straightforward way through some useful research and evaluation tools and ideas.

The book concludes with a final chapter from me where I consider some of the main themes raised, picking up on and contemplating some of the key topics and ideas, concluding by offering some handy hints and tips.

What kind of support do people facing death need?

This is an important question for all of us working in, or interested in working in, end of life care to ask. There is sometimes an assumption that the knowledge and set of skills that we learn as part of our professional training are justification enough to be employed within organisations offering health and social care services. My experiences have taught me that this can be a dangerous hypothesis. What we are able to offer needs to be useful in a number of different ways and for a number of different reasons. Of course, we must be competent enough to deliver a professional service which is of value. Nonetheless, this needs to be done by taking into account not just our own needs and those of the professional groups to which we belong, but also the needs of the people who regularly utilise services as part of their care, and more important, the needs of the organisations who provide those services and the bodies who fund them to do so.

You will read much about these kinds of issues throughout this book. However, we do offer a set of practical and positive perspectives and solutions, and individual practitioners share how they have found different ways of addressing such issues both successfully and creatively.

Some areas for consideration

Many innovative ideas and projects are also included throughout. These provide the reader with some useful exemplars of how the changing requirements of people facing the end of life, of the organisations who provide care, and of the funders and of the policy-makers alike, can be addressed and brought together by flexible and creative arts and therapies practitioners who are able, willing and motivated to constantly remould and remodel their craft in order to respond proactively and effectively to a complex range of different stressors.

Although many areas of development and innovation are shared, there are four areas that are worth considering upfront as a backdrop to some of the central chapters. These are:

1. Changing attitudes towards hospices, death and dying

2. Supporting care homes and older people

3. Creating and sustaining partnerships

4. Therapy and creating legacies.

1. Changing attitudes towards hospices, death and dying

Over the past five years, there has been an increasing drive to engage communities in talking about death and dying (see www.dyingmatters. org). At a time when the modern hospice movement in Britain was moving towards its fortieth anniversary, a BBC poll in 2006 reported that there had been little change in public attitudes towards death and dying over the past 40 years. It is now clear that this report underlined one of the major failings within the development of modern hospices.

The publication of the Department of Health's first End of Life Care Strategy in 2008 also pointed out the need to develop programmes which would challenge perceptions of death and dying in order to change public attitudes towards the end of life and to allay the fear and anxiety which occurs around death as much as is possible. The underlying aim of this imperative is not only about creating a society which is more at ease with the inevitability of death, but to create a society where the deaths of individual citizens are made better, due to advanced planning, open conversations and an overall challenging of denial and fear.

Almost ten years ago at St Christopher's, pre-empting the Department of Health's 2008 call for action, an innovative and health-promoting 'Schools Project' was formulated and piloted. This was initially devised to bring groups of adults and their carers facing the end of life together with young children and young people between the of 10 and 18. The main reason for the project is two-fold. Firstly, to change the attitudes of the young children and young people when they are at an age where this is likely to impact on their future experiences of death and dying. Secondly, for this change of attitude to be led by people who were going through the dying process themselves, enabling them to share direct experiences, educate young people, and to regain a sense of 'normality' as part of the activity. It is not the intention that those of us providing the care lead the project, rather placing the people we are caring for at the centre of it, empowering them to be in control and to share their knowledge, information and expertise for the development and good of the communities within which they live.

There are other aims, of course, such as wanting to base the project within the day care setting, in order to challenge a concept of day care which has established itself over a number of years, and rather than reiterating the experience of 'hiding away' and 'over-pampering' dying people, furnish them with the potential of retaining as much independence and influence as possible. We also want to break down some physical barriers that have been built between end of life providers and communities by unwittingly removing death and dying primarily into buildings that have come to represent fear for many individuals and the general public.

Artists and therapists have been central to the success and the development of this project and over 40 different schools within the St Christopher's catchment area have now benefitted from being involved. The creative arts continue to provide a context where children and those living with death and dying on a daily basis can come together with ease to address some difficult and complicated issues. Whether groups create a series of 'death masks' from different cultures, whether they mould clay pots to hold ashes following a cremation, or whether individual life stories are shared and transformed into performance as theatre or written into song, the creative arts have proved a useful and dynamic framework and assume a major responsibility for the projects' on-going success. Without the use of the arts, it is likely that people's fear of death and dying might not have been challenged so directly and creatively.

The project has also been rolled out in many other hospices and organisations across the UK over the years, as well as being developed in a number of other countries across the world, such as Australia, Germany and Sweden. A detailed guide to undertaking the project is available from www.stchristophers.org.uk.

In many ways this project has acted as a catalyst for further changes and developments around community engagement and end of life care. For example, St Christopher's Hospice is now open to the public. The development of the Anniversary Centre, a new day and outpatient facility, which you will also read about later in the book, is open 13 hours a day 7 days a week. Although the central purpose of the centre is to provide a growing range of services for those people who are facing death together with their friends and families, anyone from the local community is welcome to utilise the centre café, the information area and engage in a number of events and activities which bring them into close contact with dying people and those who care for them. It is important to acknowledge that artists and therapists have played a large part in enabling these more public events and activities to take place. A large, successful community choir made up of patients, carers, staff, volunteers and members of the local community meet weekly to sing together; a quilting project offers another kind of activity, as does a curry and art night and a regular professional concert series. Sunday lunches with live music bring into the building patients and families, some of whom use it as a manageable way to visit and see the hospice for the first time, together with a growing number of local older people who value a rare social opportunity to come together with others. A recent weekly initiative, 'Death Chat at St Christopher's', offers a more direct way of bringing a diverse group of people together and engaging them in conversations about death, dying and bereavement over cheese and wine. Our artists and therapists have led and supported the development of this challenging programme, which is also now motivating other similar organisations to open themselves up more effectively and enthusiastically.

For anyone wishing to work in end of life care, it will be important to articulate and demonstrate how your professional craft might support the development of such a health-promoting approach to the end of life.

2. Supporting care homes and older people

It has been clear for some time that good quality end of life care needs to be available in a range of different settings and delivered by a range of different professionals and volunteers. A growing ageing population continues to place stresses on the utilisation of good health and social care services and we all have a responsibility to explore and examine how we will be able to utilise our professional skills and personal attributes to care for older people approaching death. The Gold Standards Framework (Hansford and Meeham 2007) provides a structure to develop and support the competence and confidence of care and residential home staff, providing them with the skill and assurance to care for residents as they come to die.

Alongside good personal and nursing care, older people coming to the end of their lives in a care home also require support to tell their story, to create legacies and to discover meaning as well as to help put right difficult relationships and family rifts. We have discovered that a short programme of the creative arts and therapies can transform the experiences of older people living in care homes, motivating them to engage actively in relationships and to remain connected with others for longer.

This care and residential home programme works on a number of levels:

- Through offering a series of groups for care home residents together with staff and volunteers – these groups mainly focus on capturing people's life stories and creating legacies in the form of a range of artwork exhibitions.

- Through offering a version of the St Christopher's Schools Project in order to challenge and change attitudes towards older people and to instil a sense of responsibility into communities around caring for and about the ageing population. This is done through bringing care and residential homes together with a range of community groups such as schools, churches and pubs, in structured, short-term projects.

- Through offering teaching and support sessions for care and residential home staff, particularly activity co-ordinators, giving away knowledge and skills so that such work can be sustained into the future.

The creative arts and therapies therefore continue to support our aims and drive to change the nature of how older people are cared for and come to die within care and residential homes. It will be important for anyone wishing to work within end of life care to articulate and prove the usefulness of their specialist skill within such settings. It will also be essential to show how such specialist skills can be passed on effectively to enable those people who consistently and tirelessly work alongside older people to do so creatively and with authority.

3. Creating and sustaining partnerships

Hospices, or any other end of life care organisations, can no longer continue to provide care in silos. It is clear that the end of life care needs of many are being ineffectively met or not met at all. Although on one level, hospices have certainly developed a gold standard of what care of the dying might look like, it could also be argued that they have created problems which now require creative solutions. These problems include the downsides of looking after only a small number of people, and that the services that they provide could be viewed as expensive and too specialised. However, hospices do hold a specific set of expertise and knowledge, which can be helpful to others when reaching out to work in partnership in order to provide good care to a larger group of people at much less cost. There are many examples of organisations coming together in order to work more effectively at scale. Hospice mergers, new business models and enterprises show us different and new ways forward for the good of all those who need caring for towards the end of life.

The creative arts and therapies have enabled a number of useful and valuable partnerships to be created for the benefits of the organisation and those who use the services it provides. Partnerships with care homes, schools and other hospices and community groups as well as a range of arts organisations are mentioned throughout the book and examples of the efficacy of such innovations are shared.

One particular recent partnership project has been created between St Christopher's and the Royal Academy of Arts in London. This Project is based around a major gallery exhibition, to date Manet's 'Portraying Life' exhibition in 2013 and Hockney's 'Personal Landscapes' exhibition in 2012, and addresses a number of key issues through:

- offering a way of valuing art created by dying patients and their carers by exhibiting it alongside the work of world renowned artists at the Royal Academy of Arts

- offering a way for those people facing the end of life to discover meaning and purpose in what is happening to them through creating legacies and sharing their stories

- offering a way for dying people to stay motivated and connected to society

- offering a unique platform for the hospice and the work that it does, displaying the significance of the physical, social, psychological and spiritual needs of those people who are dying.

Workshops take place both at the hospice and at the Royal Academy of Arts, with the work created also being exhibited in both venues. To date, the project has ended with an event at the Academy, where key people, including patients and their carers, come together to debate the significance of the arts as part of both their living and dying. The work created challenges society to think differently about what it means to be dying, again shifting perceptions and changing attitudes. Ideas for creating such partnerships should be the bread and butter of the work of a creative artist or therapist within the health and social care arena. They can offer a dynamic and cost-effective way to meet some less obvious strategic imperatives as well as showing the tangible benefits that such work can bring to the organisation, to those who use its services, and to those who live within the wider community.

4. Therapy and creating legacies

The reader of this book might think that there is an underlying motive to undermine the importance of the psychotherapeutic aspects and possibilities that the creative arts and other therapies can bring to the table. It is true to say that my experience has taught me more of the value of the act of creating and being together with others rather than interpreting the psychological meaning and interpretation of what is happening for the individual. This is also true of the value and importance of the product that is created together, particularly in the form of leaving a legacy behind for others. However, I absolutely believe that there is a place to support some people at the end of their lives through intensive therapeutic support and intervention.

Two case studies: 'Listening and awareness' and 'Our music'

As a practising music therapist for many years, my main drive was to work with as many individual people who were dying as possible; I valued gaining as much experience as possible. Over the years, I worked with numerous individuals, seeing many of them only for one meeting before they died. I learned much about the benefits of using co-improvised music and I struggled to hone a language which could begin to articulate what I was learning. I have realised that the key to such work lies in what is created between, and together with, the artist or therapist and person utilising the services that we offer. I remember one gentleman referred to me by his psychologist, who told him to have some music therapy in order to unlock and to let out all of his anger. He came to meet with me and for a number of weeks bashed and crashed the percussion instruments with a set of hard sticks. His playing could be described as extremely loud and mainly chaotic. There was no acknowledgement from him in any way that I was attempting to play along with him, and I doubt that he could have heard me among all the noise that he was making. A few weeks into working together something happened. I still have the tape recording of our improvisations, and there is a moment when his music and my music connect directly – he listens to himself and to me for the first time and hears something. He is visibly shocked and responds by stopping playing immediately: 'This is not about me letting out all my anger is it?' he asks (pause)… 'it's about you and me doing something together and doing something that makes sense. I wondered why you were here as I could make a loud noise and let out all of my anger all by myself without you…now I know that it's about both of us creating something together…' Another person who I worked with loved improvising operatic arias while I accompanied. Following one intensive improvisation, the person offered the following explanation:

> You know my body is fading away by the day, the 'outside' of me is dying. When we improvise the focus is on the 'inside', the inside of me is living and when we play it grows and expands… We have two very clear things; I refer to these as 'your' music and 'my' music. Initially we are separate and then almost always, something special happens. Then what we have is what I would call 'our music'. Here we are totally one, totally equal, in balance. During these times there is no illness, I am completely well; in fact, I never felt so alive… (Hartley 2000, p.109)

Other such stories are also shared throughout which we hope will enable the realisation that what is created and experienced between us in this work is more expansive and valuable than what can be created alone. The uniqueness of what is created is the true value of such work and not solely the expression of the obvious vulnerability, pain and trauma of the individual.

We should always be asking ourselves 'What kind of artist, what kind of therapist, does the person who is dying or bereaved, the organisation I work for, and the wider world of health and social care need me to be?' and also 'What do I bring to the table that is unique and different from any other practitioner within the multi-disciplinary team?' It is hoped that the breadth of different projects, experiences and work shared within this book will go some way to revealing the variety of possible answers to these questions.

Conclusion

In 2008, I co-edited a book with Malcolm Payne called *The Creative Arts in Palliative Care* (Hartley and Payne 2008) and we ended the introduction to the book in the following way:

> We cannot yet claim that the arts are a vital force in the future of people's care when they come to die, but we can keep the arts central within the current dialogue and debate of what will constitute an holistic, efficient and cost effective package of…services for the future. (p.20)

Five years later we may not have moved on much further in claiming the vitality of the arts, therapies or arts therapies for people who are living with death and dying. However, needing to justify this work in this way may no longer be so crucial, as it does seem somewhat clearer that the argument should not necessarily now be around the efficacy of the creative arts or therapies, but about how the more confident and competent artist or therapist himself chooses to utilise and articulate his craft in a variety of ways, for a range of different reasons and to meet a number of strategic challenges.

The future lies not only in the breadth of possibilities and experiences that the creative arts and therapies may or may not offer, but in the creative practitioner's ability to utilise his skills and knowledge flexibly and openly in order to respond to the challenges and changes that we face in the world of health and social care today. One other issue important for the artist or therapist to consider is what the financial cost of a flexible and competent artist or therapist should be. It remains to be seen whether the regulation and registration of the arts therapies and other therapy professions will, in fact, lead to them, out of necessity, being priced out of the health and social care market place. During times of financial uncertainty, we must remind ourselves that it is possible, and probably necessary, to be flexible and competitive on financial cost and also that it is reasonable, on occasion, to be able to offer some time and expertise for free, particularly if tendering something new and different. My experience has shown that a 'test and learn' model has both the potential and possibility to pay dividends in the long term.

The cost effective, flexible and creative practitioner is therefore of more value to the current health and social care sector than the one who remains rigid within the sometimes narrow parameters imposed on his work by the educational establishment where he has trained or by the professional discipline to which he belongs.

References

Hansford, P. and Meeham, H. (2007) Gold Standards Framework: Improving community care. Available at www.endoflifejournal.stchristophers.org.uk/.../gold-standards-framework, accessed on 10 October 2012.

Hartley, N. (2000) 'Musiktherapie mit menschen, Die mit HIV und AIDS leben: "…Beinahe die definition Gottes…"' In I.V. Kairos, *Beirtrage zur Musiktherapie in der Medzin Hrsg*. David Aldridge. Nern, Gottingen, Toronto, Seattle: Verlag Hans Huber.

Hartley, N. and Payne, M. (2008) *The Creative Arts in Palliative Care*. London and Philadelphia, PA: Jessica Kingsley Publishers.

Chapter 2

The Model and Philosophy of Hospice and End of Life Care

Introduction

This chapter outlines some of the history and gives a view of the model and philosophy of the modern hospice movement and end of life care. A short biography of Cicely Saunders is given and her original vision is discussed, including her formation of the concept of 'total pain', as well as brief introductions to how it has been translated in different ways across the world. Important areas such as multi-disciplinary working are briefly introduced and information about funding mechanisms of services is presented. Part of the chapter focuses on articulating and understanding the philosophical components of good end of life care from my own personal experience. The chapter ends with two case studies, concentrating on some of the main themes previously highlighted.

The following headings are used to focus on some of the key issues:

- Dame Cicely Saunders: a short biography

- Total pain

- The multi-disciplinary team

- Care, education and research

- St Christopher's today

- National and international agencies

- Funding mechanisms, fundraising and budgets

- Funding: an international perspective

- End of life care: what lies at the heart?

- Two case studies

- Final thoughts.

Dame Cicely Saunders: a short biography

Cicely Saunders was born in 1918 and died at St Christopher's Hospice, London in 2005. In 1938 Saunders attended St Anne's College, Oxford to read politics, philosophy and economics, as her parents had disapproved of her interest in studying nursing. In 1940, after the beginning of the Second World War, she took a break from her studies to train in nursing at the Nightingale School for Nursing based at St Thomas's Hospital, London. Following a serious back problem which had troubled her since childhood, in 1944 she was unable to continue a nursing career so she returned to St Anne's College, Oxford in 1945 and completed a war degree. She went on to train as a hospital almoner, again at St Thomas's Hospital, London (Monroe 2008).

One of Saunders' peculiarities was her openness in talking about the relationships that she formed with some of the patients under her care. In 1948, while working as an almoner at London's Archway Hospital, she formed a relationship with a Polish immigrant, David Tasma, who having escaped Nazi Germany and the Warsaw ghetto came to London where he had worked as a waiter. Tasma was one of three Polish men who were to be significant to her at different stages of her life. At the time she met him, Saunders was working as an almoner and she frequently visited him while he was dying of cancer. They spoke together of creating a place where those coming to the end of their life could be allowed to do so with hope and dignity. He bequeathed her £500 which was to be 'a window in your home'. This inspired Saunders to begin to formulate the vision which would eventually become St Christopher's Hospice, the first purpose-built modern hospice in the world. This donation and her debt to Tasma are now commemorated on a simple memorial plaque which sits beneath a large plain glass window at the front of the hospice in South East London.

While training as a medical social worker, Saunders met a group of Christians and was converted to the Christian faith. This faith would remain central to her life and work until she died. At the end of the 1940s, she began working part-time at St Luke's Home for the Poor in Bayswater and in 1957 qualified as a doctor, understanding from a surgeon called Dr Barrett that if she was going to realise her vision of creating a place where dying could be seen as a normal experience and managed well, she would have more influence and clout if she was a medical practitioner.

A year later, she began working at the Roman Catholic St Joseph's Hospice for the dying poor in Hackney, East London, where she remained for seven years. It was here that she began her early research into pain and symptom control. While working at St Joseph's, she met another Polish patient, Antoni Michniewicz. His death in 1960 further inspired her to set up her own hospice. Saunders gained the support of a number of key, influential people, who understood and bought into her vision (Clark 2002).

In 1980, Saunders married the Polish artist Marian Bohusz-Szyszko after a long friendship which had begun in 1963. A few years later, she bought a copy of one of his large religious works which was to be hung within the hospice. It is not insignificant that he set up an art studio within St Christopher's where he practised for many years. Saunders was made a Dame of the Order of the British Empire in 1980 and received the honour of Order of Merit in 1989. Marian Bohusz-Szyszko died at the hospice in 1995 and Saunders outlived him by ten years, dying herself at St Christopher's in July 2005 (Monroe 2008).

Most hospices, both in the UK and abroad, will have their story. The story might involve entrepreneurial individuals who used their energy and expertise to motivate a community of people to set up the organisation. These stories will be seen to be important, as in many ways, they form the foundation for the organisational culture and behaviour. It might be important to understand the hospice story if you are contemplating going to work for it. More information is given about starting out in a new job within a hospice in Chapter 9, 'Getting Started'.

Total pain

There were, of course, other hospices before St Christopher's. These hospices were centres of dedicated nursing care for the terminally ill, but they were not what we now think of as modern palliative care (Baines 2011). St Christopher's Hospice, London was officially opened in 1967 and is widely thought to be the 'first modern hospice'. What is meant by this is that it was the first purpose-built centre where people and their families could come to be cared for as they were dying with the support of a team committed to pain and symptom management with in-depth psychological, social and spiritual support. Saunders (1988) defined this concept as 'total pain' and this was later adapted and defined by the World Health Organization (WHO) as follows (see MacLeod 2007; see also www.socrates.org/mod/page/view.php?id=13276):

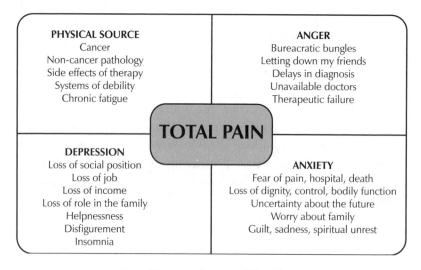

Figure 2.1: Total pain as defined by the
World Health Organization (WHO)

The multi-disciplinary team

It was always Saunders' intention that this support mechanism for delivering the 'total pain' package be delivered by a multi-disciplinary team, as providing care in this way was more than one person could ever deliver alone (Baines 2011), this team which would include doctors, nurses, physiotherapists, social workers, chaplains and others and the focus would be to share knowledge, skills and values for the benefit of patients and their families (Speck 2006). Chapter 4 focusses more closely on what it is like from the artist's or therapist's perspective to work as part of a multi-disciplinary team. St Christopher's Hospice, although one of the largest in the UK with a workforce of over 300 staff, is typical in terms of the professions it employs to make up the multi-disciplinary team. Figure 2.2 outlines one version of how the multi-disciplinary team might look:

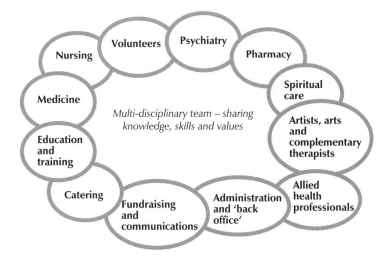

Figure 2.2: An example of a multi-disciplinary team

It is vital that teams learn how to share, and experience sharing, their knowledge, skills and values. Peter Speck lists some of the important values of multi-disciplinary teamwork (2006):

- the importance of working together to achieve the aim

- each team member deserves respect

- open and honest communication

- open access to information.

Living out these values on a day to day basis is not straightforward. It demands commitment from individual members of the team. One of the challenges for multi-disciplinary working at the current time is the complexity of responding to the needs of many staff to work part-time or flexible hours. This provides problems with attendance at regular multi-disciplinary team meetings where values should be shared, practised and accomplished. This means that the input from some professionals cannot impact effectively either onto the professional team or, more important, into the patient's care. This will be the case for many artists or therapists working in hospice or end of life care today, as it is unlikely that many of these types of roles will be full-time positions. Another difficulty for the multi-disciplinary team will be the need to understand and engage with a plethora of individualised professional languages (Hartley 2011). Professional discourse within specific professions will be more advanced in some than others. For example, the language used by medicine might be more accepted and understood than the language used by artists or some therapists. It may, therefore, be important to be able to challenge any assumptions or hierarchical difficulties that might arise because of this. Understanding each other's professional discourse will be vital if every profession is to be accepted and valued as a part of the team. It is important to take this seriously when beginning any work in end of life care, and to take time to learn about and appreciate the possibilities, but also complexities, that this might bring.

Care, education and research

Saunders' vision was based not only on providing high quality care in a place where people's dying could be treated as a normal process and managed well, but on utilising the experiences gained at St Christopher's to teach and influence others, particularly those working in the National Health Service (NHS) from where she gained her early experiences (Monroe and Oliviere 2003).

Care and education were linked to her quest to understand what worked and did not work through an intense programme of research and evaluation. Some of Saunders' and her team's early research challenged the very heart of medicine. Saunders had noticed through her earlier work in the NHS, that management of pain was based on the patient actually being in pain before any pain control could be given. Saunders and her peers' early research at St Christopher's proved that the use of moderate doses of strong opiates at regular intervals could control and manage people's pain a lot more effectively. An outcry from the medical establishment accused her of creating a dependency on drugs which might be seen as unethical (Clark 1999; Twycross 1974).

In 1987, Palliative Medicine was formally recognised as a medical speciality, and over 40 years since its inception, Saunders' trinity of care, education and research still sits at the heart of the work of hospices and other end of life care units. Research and evaluation is discussed more in Chapter 11.

St Christopher's today

St Christopher's is currently one of the largest of around 300 hospices and specialist palliative care units in the UK, and as a result of its history holds a significant local, national and international reputation; there are also end of life care initiatives in over 115 countries. As a local community provision, it serves a population of 1.5 million people across South East London, incorporating the London Boroughs of Bromley, Southwark, Lewisham, Lambeth and Croydon. St Christopher's is a registered charity and costs around £17 million a year to run. It receives around a third of its costs from the NHS, with the rest of its income generated from other areas including legacies, voluntary donations and fundraising. The building houses a 48-bedded inpatient unit, and a day care and outpatient service, known as the Anniversary Centre. Also, on any one day staff will be providing medical, nursing, social, psychological and supportive care to over 850 patients and those who care for them within the places that they live. A purpose-built education centre attracts around 4000 students on-site every year with a further 3000 students being reached through outreach education programmes. The education centre runs about 70 training courses each year including an MSc in Palliative care run jointly with King's College, London and Diplomas in both child and adult bereavement accredited by Middlesex University (Monroe 2008).

National and international agencies

From a national and international perspective, and as the hospice movement developed, initially across the UK and then throughout the rest of the world, Help the Hospices (HtH) was set up in 1986 and their offices are based in London. This organisation is a charity and provides representation and support and guidance to hospices across the UK and offers information and advice to other countries across the world, especially if they want to set up an end of life care service in a new geographical area. More recently it has become a membership organisation (www.helpthehospices.org.uk).

The National Council for Palliative Care (NCPC) was formed in 1991 and describes itself as the umbrella charity for all those involved in palliative, end of life and hospice care in England, Wales and Northern Ireland. The council takes a leading role in working with the Department of Health and the NHS acting as a single body which speaks on behalf of end of life care service providers (www.ncpc.org. uk).

The European Association for Palliative Care (EAPC) was established in 1988, with 42 founding members. The aim of the EAPC is to promote palliative care in Europe and to act as a focus for all of those who work, or have an interest, in the field of palliative care at the scientific, clinical and social levels. It organises a bi-annual congress which has the major aim of bringing together end of life care practitioners from across Europe in order to share experiences and learn from each other, while obtaining the best media coverage possible in order to spread information about the EAPC and palliative care. The EAPC also acts as a research hub, providing opportunities for individuals and organisations to come together in order to examine new initiatives (www.eapcnet.eu).

The International Association for Hospice and Palliative Care (IAHPC) was set up in the 1980s to encourage and enable each country across the world, according to its resources and conditions, to develop its own model of palliative care provision. The association focuses on programme development, education, information dissemination and policy changes to improve availability of good and adequate care of patients with advanced diseases (www.hospicecare.com).

Many of the countries which have been influenced by, and have developed a commitment to Saunders' vision of high quality end of life care will have their own national professional groups and leaders. For example, Florence Wald (1917–2008) was a nurse and dean of the Yale School of Nursing in the USA. Her early interest in and contact with Saunders inspired her to become a pioneer in the development of systems for the delivery of end of life care across the USA (Adams 2010). Similarly in Canada, Dr Balfour Mount (b. 1939) visited St Christopher's and worked alongside Saunders in the early 1970s. His visit, along with his study of the work of Kubler-Ross (1969), inspired him to open the first end of life care ward in Montreal's Royal Victoria Hospital. He is also accredited with coining the term 'palliative care' (2003).

Examples of other national groups and associations include Hospice New Zealand (www.hospice.org.nz) which was formulated in 1986, the Indian Association of Palliative Care (www.palliativecare. in) which was established in 1994, and the African Palliative Care Association (APCA) founded in 2004 (www.africanpalliativecare.org).

Funding mechanisms, fundraising and budgets

In the UK, end of life care delivered by hospices has always been free at the point of delivery and remains so to this day. Most hospices are fairly small independent charities with a loyalty to local communities and the need to engage financial support from them (Hartley and Payne 2008).

Over 40 years since the birth of the modern hospice movement, at a time of unprecedented global recession, the NHS has accepted its duty to offer its users a quality end of life care (EOLC) service. At a time of significant financial pressure, the first *End of Life Care Strategy* was published by the Department of Health in July 2008. It highlights the following as key to future successful delivery of quality end of life care:

- emphasis on disparity – quality EOLC for all conditions, in all settings, with an absolute focus on community provision

- emphasis on a 'whole systems' approach – linking up health and social care agencies and skilling up generalist providers through tools and frameworks

- emphasis on new money being available for new services which will be locally commissioned

- emphasis on developing a national EOLC intelligence network and developing the responsibility of the National Coalition on EOLC

- emphasis on identifying dying, culture change, co-ordinated assessment, care planning and developing communication skills

- emphasis on developing rapid response 24/7 services.

How this growing demand and pressure for good end of life care for all can be achieved with a decreasing number of resources, while moving into a new competitive market place, where the emphasis will probably be focussed more on cost rather than quality, will continue to be a complicated predicament for the established hospice movement (Monroe 2008).

Initially, it appeared that rather than focus on developing service delivery in preparation for the new Department of Health strategy, many UK hospices focussed on defending their patch, arguing that what they provide needs no change, while continuing to put pressure on primary care trusts (PCTs) for increased funding. This pressure for increased funding, and in some cases for funding parity with the statutory sector, has impelled the NHS to demand an evaluated, comprehensive, cost effective service delivery model from hospices with a focus on outcomes, based on them finding solutions rather than problems (Monroe 2008).

I have already mentioned that the first donation towards the building of St Christopher's Hospice came in the form of £500 from Saunders' patient, David Tasma – '…I will be a window in your home…' This act was the beginning of how charity would become important, and remain important, to the majority of modern hospices, particularly within the United Kingdom. Hospice care within the UK was set up as a protest against the 'death denial' of the new National Health Service of the 1950s, and although it was Saunders' intention to influence end of life care within the NHS as the years went by, the hospice movement remains on the periphery of the NHS system. On the one hand, this provides most modern hospices with the possibility of registering as charities with the freedom and independence to find money through fundraising. This extra income could explain the 'added extras' provided by independent hospices such as day care services, quality care to families and loved ones and extensive bereavement support. Most hospices in the UK will now receive some financial income from the NHS via what are known currently as primary care trusts. However there is an inequity of support from PCTs across the country, with hospices receiving anywhere between 10 per cent and 60 per cent towards their annual cost base. Disparity lies at the heart of current challenges for end of life care and this is not only restricted to funding. The lack of a consistent national approach to the delivery of 24/7 end of life care, highlighted as an essential baseline of care within the *End of Life Care Strategy*, presents another shortfall for current service providers. Current strategic challenges are explored in more detail in Chapter 3.

At the time of writing, a palliative care funding review (Hughes-Hallett, Craft and Davies 2010) is being undertaken within the UK and the outcome is uncertain. We wait to hear if the review will, in the first instance, bring a greater equity of financial support to hospices across the country, or if the business will become tougher through opening the possibility of new private providers being encouraged into the market place and potential competition between hospices.

This being the case, hospices will find themselves within a competitive market place for the first time in their history.

Taking St Christopher's as an example, at the present time it costs around £17 million to run each year. Roughly, a third of this comes from the PCTs or the new clinical commissioning groups (CCGs), with around a third coming from legacies, and another third coming from a variety of fundraising endeavours. At a time of global recession, challenges are present in all three of these areas. As well as the move to commissioning of services from PCTs/CCGs to general practitioners (GPs) themselves, one of the big questions at the present moment, particularly with regard to the UK funding review, is what kind of things should society pay for? The government is in the process of deciding what package of care people coming to the end of their life really need from the 'state'. It is likely that this will include core services such as nursing and medicine, leaving the more 'peripheral' provisions to be funded by the general public. This is important, particularly for artists and therapists who are thinking of pursuing a career in end of life care. It will be unlikely that many posts will be funded from statutory sources; funding will need to be found elsewhere. In many ways, it is good to know this, as it may very well be a waste of time and energy lobbying and attempting to persuade the government to fund professions that it does not have the resources or perceived responsibility to support.

Funding: an international perspective

Although the hospice movement has spread throughout the world, it has done so with national and cultural imperatives and differences in mind. It is clear that in some countries, resistance to the values and practice of palliative care has, for instance, sprung from both cultural and religious factors which have included the difficulties of talking openly about death and dying, the fear of failure from the medical profession, and the inability to accept new and different medical procedures and techniques such as the availability of opioids. Funding mechanisms in different countries will have been adopted and moulded according to a range of different key factors. As mentioned, cultural and religious differences will have been influential, as will the national systems and structures that have been developed to fund health and social care across the board.

For example, in the USA, most medical care is provided as part of personal insurance plans. Most hospice care is provided in the home and is also available to people in nursing homes, assisted living facilities, veterans' facilities, hospitals and prisons (Connor 2007–2008). Medicare, a private insurance provider, includes the provision of medicines, equipment, 24/7 access to care, and offers bereavement support following a death.

In Canada, the model of care developed by Mount following his visit to St Christopher's Hospice, was more focussed towards a hospital-based approach. This focus was motivated, and the delivery of end of life care services was modelled, by the different funding mechanisms in Canada as opposed to the UK (Hamilton 1995). Nevertheless, despite the prominence of palliative care in Canada, which has one of the largest and best established congresses in the world taking place every two years, in 2004, it was stated that palliative care was only available to between 5 and 15 per cent of all Canadians, and services were continuing to decrease due to cuts in government funding (CHPCA 2002). It is also stated that the majority of Canada's ten provinces did not identify palliative care as a core health service.

End of life care: what lies at the heart?

It is well documented that Cicely Saunders was strongly guided by her Christian faith when setting up the model of care at St Christopher's which was to transform care of the dying across the world. However, at the heart of this phenomenon lies a very human response to the suffering and vulnerability of others. The statement made by Saunders, '…you matter because you are you and you matter to the last moment of your life…we will do all we can, not only to help you die peacefully, but to live until you die…' (Clark 2002), lies at the centre of any simple inquiry into the model that she created. Of course, the statement highlights that every human being is unique and has the right to be treated so up until the point of death; there is also the promise that the model will aspire to help people live their dying without pain and undue fear, remaining conscious enough to partake still in the stuff of life. However, it is important not just to take this statement at a superficial level. It could be said that Saunders is setting down a direct challenge. Is she really saying that no matter who the dying person is, that regardless of what they have done or who they have been in their life, they will be welcomed and treated the same as the next person? This challenge goes beyond the everyday prejudices of race, colour or creed, beyond what people believe and practice, and hits right into the centre of human behaviour and personality. Most of us in our lives will find the practices and activities of some other human beings indefensible and personally repulsive. The important question for those of us engaged in this work, is what kind of person will press our button? Who will we find it difficult to welcome and treat well as stated within Saunders' philosophical remit? A murderer, a burglar or a paedophile? A rapist, a fraudster or a bully? Because someone finds themselves dying, this does not mean they will become, or even strive to become, a reformed character. And yet, our commitment, according to Saunders, is to welcome them in and treat them, not only well, but with humility and unconditional human kindness. This is indeed a big ask, a complex and demanding mission. Key to accepting people as they are is developing the craft of 'getting ourselves out of the way'.

Paying attention: giving a good impression

Most of us in our lives are experts in giving a good impression that we are paying attention; we do it every day of our lives and we do it well. The three tools used to listen well are normally stated as follows:

1. body language

2. eye contact

3. active listening.

If we position our body in a certain way, use eye contact with the person we are with, and nod or shake our head at appropriate moments, we are said to be good listeners. But is this really the case? An example might be that if we are with a patient we have met a number of times before, and they begin telling us the same story that we have heard a number of times before, our personal feelings can get in the way. What I mean by this is that we can hold our body in a certain way, nod in all the appropriate moments and make direct eye contact, because we know what the structure of the story is already. The tools can be used to great effect, but in reality, in my mind, I can be planning what I am going to do later in the day. Here, I would be using my expertise of 'giving a good impression' that I am paying attention. This is what most of us do very well, not because we are not good listeners or communicators, but because on the whole, the way that most of us listen is less than average. Martin Buber writes:

> ...the help that human beings give each other in becoming a self, leads the life between them to its height... (Buber 1937, p.22)

This 'life between' offers the potential and possibility for something to happen between us in the relationships that we have. Saunders talks about getting to the 'right depth of regard' (Saunders 1988) and Marie De Hennezel talks of the distance required in order to meet with someone effectively and respectfully (De Hennezel 1998). I would like to suggest that this depth, or distance, or 'life between' offers the space for us within which to do our job well. Here, I would like to introduce a three-level model of paying attention.

Paying attention: three levels

It is possible that personal feelings can be acknowledged and put to one side, in order that we can pay attention and respond appropriately to whatever, or whoever, is before our eyes. Simone Weil, in a book called *Waiting for God* (Weil 1951) writes: 'those who are unhappy have no need for anything else in this world apart from someone who is capable of giving them their attention'.

In terms of responding to other people, my understanding is that we respond on three different levels:

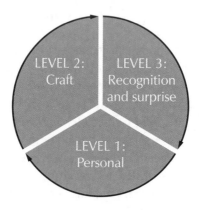

Figure 2.3: Three levels of listening (Hartley 2005)

Level 1: the personal response

When we meet someone for the first time, most of us will respond on a personal level. This first level of response is the most straightforward and easily recognisable. The engagement with another human being will bring up for us personal feelings. How many of us will have met someone for the first time, and before speaking with them, or knowing any facts about them, will have made an instant judgement? 'I don't like that person' or 'I'd like to get to know that person' will be common responses. This is because we will be responding from a personal perspective. This may be to do with what the person looks like, or if they remind us of someone else we have known in the past. These feelings, although in many cases based on a learned instinct, can get in the way of us being of help or use to the other person. When we have a role to play of welcoming or helping the person to know themselves as important or special, we need to step aside from these initial responses and simply do our job.

Level 2: using our craft

Craft is a word not often used in our modern day lives. My grandmother spoke of certain people of her generation learning their craft; this may have been as a blacksmith, a baker or a seamstress. This notion of craft, I believe, can be defined as the set of skills, or how we bring together the various bits of stuff, that we need to do our job effectively. Utilising this stuff and marrying it well with the set of skills we have can bring our craft to the height of its powers. Craft might be utilised in the making of a cup of tea and giving it to someone in a certain way that helps them to feel noticed and served well; it may well be the way that we pay attention and notice certain key points of detail that are troubling the person resulting in anxiety and disruption; it might be the way that we combine certain medicines in order to understand and alleviate a person's unique set of medical symptoms. Whatever it is, done well, it can change lives and provide a way of separating our personal feelings from the act of helping another human being. To put it simply, in order to use our craft well, we must first of all learn to be able to get ourselves out of the way.

Level 3: recognition and surprise

Sometimes, the ability to utilise our craft competently and well can be surprising, both to ourselves and to those we care for. Recognition and surprise will probably come at the moment when something is going well, or when we reach new unexpected peaks as part of the work that we do. For a therapist, this might come at a time when focussing on a particular familiar problem which has up until this moment seemed unmoveable and a constant challenge. Suddenly there is freedom and movement, a realisation, or a new understanding. At these moments, using an internal narrative we will sometimes take time to be pleased with ourselves and those with whom we are working or to ask ourselves how have we managed such a thing, why did we do it, what did we do differently and how did it come about?

There is a strong link between the personal level and these moments of surprise. The real irony is that in order to digest both of these experiences, we need to withdraw inside of ourselves, albeit sometimes momentarily, in order to process them; in real terms, we have to stop paying attention, stop using our craft and we become removed, removed enough to stop focussing on what we are doing and on what needs to be done next.

In actuality, we do not move effortlessly and methodically from one level to the other, and any encounter engages us in moving sporadically between the levels with no defined order. I would like to suggest that when we are intent on being of help and support to another human being, we need to be at the second level of craft as much as possible. It is on this level where we do what we do well; it is the place we inhabit in order to do our job, the place where we are able to keep that all important 'professional distance', the place where we 'get ourselves out of the way' (Mayne 1998).

Case study: paying attention and levels of awareness

When I began to work at one particular hospice, I was asked to shadow a nurse on a night shift on the inpatient ward; it is an experience that I remember vividly. In reality, I helped make hot drinks for patients, carers and staff members, I sat and held the hand of a dying patient who was alone, answered the telephone and, on the whole, I would like to think, made myself useful. It was important to see the working of the organisation in this way, and also to be thrown in at the deep end.

One of the things that I will always remember was observing a nurse changing the dressing on a patient's facial tumour. It was explained to the patient that I was a new member of staff and I am sure that I was asked in order to be another pair of hands, to help make sure that the patient was as comfortable as possible during the process, rather than for any well thought out educational purpose. However, educational it certainly was. I sat alongside the patient as the nurse went through the process of removing the dressing, cleaning and tidying up the wound, and reapplying a fresh, clean dressing.

My first memory was of being overwhelmed by a pungent, offensive odour coming from the wound; the second was a repulsion towards the physicality of the wound itself. This 'Level 1' response almost overpowered me. Everything inside of myself was telling me to run and to retreat in horror from the room. How the nurse was bearing it I could not imagine.

As I began to focus on what the nurse was doing, the horror withdrew from my mind and I found myself transfixed by the detail of her work. The care, consideration and attention to detail was riveting and demanded my complete attention. I realised that she was able to bear it because she was doing her job. The 'stuff' of her job was so well-honed, and her commitment to doing it in the best possible way was almost palpable. The patient was calm, accepting and respected throughout.

After the dressing was complete and we had left the room, I asked the nurse how she had managed to do the dressing, when the odour and visual impact of the wound were so strong. She told me that there was no point getting caught up in things like that. She said that she had a job to do and if she did not do it how else was it going to get done?

This story is a good example of being able to get ourselves out of the way in order to be of service to others. Observing the excellence of the nurse's craft instilled in me a certain level of confidence. As she got her personal responses and reactions out of the way and focussed on the job in hand, the very thing that she did well helped focus herself, myself and I am sure, the patient, to remain fully present and, most important, accepting of the situation. Everything was dignified and respectful.

Case study: Susan

I first met Susan when she was referred to me for some music therapy by one of the medical consultants at a hospice. Susan was a white, well-to-do lady in her late sixties. She was living with an AIDS diagnosis. Susan had been attending the hospice for outpatient clinics with the consultant or a community nurse specialist for a number of months, and had declined any offer of referral into any of the other hospice services, including day care. She had lived alone since her family had disowned her when she had been diagnosed with HIV a couple of years earlier, and the only person she had regular contact with was a volunteer from the hospice who would regularly help with shopping and other practical tasks. My sense is that the medical consultant referred Susan to me mostly out of desperation. He indeed had tried a number of things in the past, which she had always refused. For whatever reason, and I still do not quite understand why, when the consultant referred her for some music therapy, Susan accepted.

I met with Susan usually once a week and this lasted over a period of about three months. She came to see me at the hospice and we spent anything from 30 to 60 minutes together. It was clear from the first time I met her, and also understandable, that Susan was depressed. My relationship with her remained, for the most part, monosyllabic. What I mean by this is that Susan never offered me any information about herself, she never once initiated a conversation or discussion, when I asked questions or spoke with her, she answered me occasionally but with only one word, and she never played a musical instrument. Our time together was spent in silence for the most part. Initially I would ask a question, or suggest that we attempt to play some music together, but she only ever responded with one-word answers, keeping her head down and making no eye contact. In many ways, it was extremely frustrating, and I remember wanting to suggest many times that she stopped coming for the sessions. I stopped myself from doing this, however, as I realised, that even if, for me, nothing seemed to be happening, she returned every week for our meeting. The simple act of her doing this each week motivated me to continue, however difficult and incomprehensible it was to spend the time with her. After all, she was making the effort to turn up, and it was not my job to judge and assume that nothing of value was happening.

When we had been meeting for almost three months, Susan was admitted to the inpatient unit of the hospice with pneumocystis pneumonia, which could be fatal for people living with AIDS. Over the days that she was in the hospice, she began to get stronger and on this particular day she came to see me in my music therapy room from her room on the ward. For the most part, our experience of being together was no different to any time previously. Susan was quiet and withdrawn and did not speak. We sat quietly together for over half an hour. At this point I said to her that we still had some time left if there was anything she wanted to talk about or do together. When I had said this in the past, we normally sat quietly for a short period and then Susan would get up and leave the room. I had just started to settle down into silence and something very unexpected occurred. Susan, completely out of the blue, started to sing. I was shocked, but found that my initial very quick and immediate response was to turn to the piano which was to my left and begin to accompany her. There were three things that shocked and surprised me:

1. That Susan started to sing in the first place.

2. When Susan sang, she just didn't sing single notes, like she had done when she had used words. Her melodic line, although with a voice shaky to start, was elongated and drawn out. She formed

complete music phrases; I had never heard her form a complete sentence.

3. The content of the words that she sang. Initially she sang non-verbally to 'Ah', but then she began to use words. The words that she used are below. In reality, I believe that she was using the situation to say goodbye to her friends and family. Although they had all disowned her, this is almost like a ritual in order to actively say goodbye to them:

(non-verbal singing – both of us)

Ah...

Oh Lord our God

Thy children call

Grant us thy peace

'til the sunrise...

Goodnight... Goodnight...

(spoken)

Keep all our family in your care,

Love us all, as we know you do.

Still, Goodnight and God bless

to friends, family and those that we love.

(Singing again)

Goodnight... Keep us in your care.

Amen... Amen.

I have discovered since that the first four lines of Susan's song are the 'Brownie's Goodnight song'; I did not know this at the time. I accompanied her gently and sang non-verbally from time to time, normally when her voice became slightly weaker, in order to encourage her to continue. Looking back at the three levels of listening mentioned earlier in the chapter, I would like to use this experience with Susan to explain some of the points raised.

Level 1: the personal response

When Susan begins to sing, my initial response, which is a personal one, is one of being shocked. In reality, I wanted Susan to stop. I was confused about what she was doing, and it all felt rather difficult.

Level 2: using our craft

When I was able to get myself to Level 2, and this happened very quickly, I began to listen to her singing 'as music'. My craft in this instance is music itself. I hear her begin to sing a 'falling minor second' – an E flat descending to a D. It seems natural then to firmly route the song in C minor. It is important to realise here that the choice of C minor as a key is not because I felt 'sad'. It is because I am responding as a musician to what I have heard as I would do to any other person singing.

Level 3: recognition and surprise

I struggled very hard to keep myself on Level 2 as much as possible. In many ways, it was the place where I was safe, as I knew what I was doing and was using my musical expertise. Of course, from time to time I was pulled back to Level 1, and then had to begin again by focussing quickly on the musical content, in order to respond with my musical craft. From time to time I also find myself on Level 3. These are the moments when I begin to be surprised by the quality of what is being created. The music is so complete, as if rehearsed, and I pause internally to either congratulate myself or to be surprised by Susan's involvement and creativity.

During both Level 1 and Level 3, I stop listening and have to continually refocus myself on being of service to her, of utilising my craft, of practising as a musician.

Final thoughts

Although some might argue that the act of 'being of service' lies at the heart of Saunders' Christian belief and ministry and was therefore essential to the formation of her vision for comprehensive and high quality end of life care, no religious faith has the monopoly on basic human kindness. It may be the case that all religions focus on the need to be considerate towards, and help out, both friends and strangers. In reality, what they do is to provide a variety of frameworks and structures which can be utilised and practised as part of their own particular philosophy and belief systems. In reality, one does not need a particular religious creed in order to be of service to others. The arts, for example, are by their very nature hospitable. They welcome people in and offer structures and frameworks to be together in good, strong and healthy ways.

The view given in this chapter of the philosophy of hospice care is a very personal one, but taken from years of experience and learning. As human beings, we should naturally aspire to help others, and to do so in 'minute particulars' (Mayne 1998). Shaping and honing our craft should not be done solely for our own personal satisfaction or for the satisfaction of others, but in order to help people who are vulnerable to experience the reality that they genuinely do matter, right up until the last moment of their life.

References

Adams, C. (2010) 'Dying with dignity in America: The transformational leadership of Florence Wald.' *Journal of Professional Nursing 26*, 2, 125–132.

Baines, M. (2011) 'Tackling Total Pain.' In C. Saunders (ed.) *Hospice and Palliative Care. An Interdisciplinary Approach* (pp.26–39). London, Melbourne, Auckland: Edward Arnold. Available at www.stchristophers.org.uk/about/history, accessed on 17 June 2013.

Buber, M. (1937) *I am Thou*. Edinburgh: T&T Clark.

CHPCA (Canadian Hospice Palliative Care Association) (2002) *A Model to Guide Hospice Palliative Care: Based on National Principles and Norms of Practice*. Ottawa, ON: CHPCA. Available at www.chpca.net/media/7422/a-model-to-guide-hospice-palliative-care-2002-urlupdate-august2005.pdf, accessed on 17 June 2013.

Clark, D. (2002) *Cicely Saunders: Founder of the Hospice Movement. Selected Letters 1959–1999*. Oxford: Oxford University Press.

Clark, D. (1999) '"Total pain," disciplinary power and the body in the work of Cicely Saunders, 1958–1967.' *Society of Scientific Medicine 49*, 6, 727–736.

Connor, S.R. (2007–2008) 'Development of hospice and palliative care in the United States.' *Omega (Westport) 56*, 1, 89–99.

De Hennezel, M. (1998) *Intimate Death*. Auckland: Warner Books.

DH (Department of Health) (2008) *The End of Life Care Strategy*. Available at www.endoflifecareforadults.nhs.uk, accessed on 17 June 2013.

Hamilton, J. (1995) 'Dr Balfour Mount and our cruel irony of our care for the dying.' *Canadian Medical Association Journal 153*, 3, 334–336.

Hartley, N. (2005) 'Love Actually – Attempting to Articulate the Heart of Hospice.' In C. Dileo and J. Loewy (eds) *Music Therapy at the End of Life*. Cherry Hill, NJ: Jeffrey Books.

Hartley, N. (2011) 'Spirituality and the Arts – Discovering what Really Matters.' In B. Rumbold (ed.) *Spirituality and Healthcare*. Oxford: Oxford University Press.

Hartley, N. and Payne, M. (2008) *The Creative Arts in Palliative Care*. London and Philadelphia, PA: Jessica Kingsley Publishers.

Hughes-Hallett, T., Craft, C. and Davies, C. (2011) *Funding Review: Funding the Right Care and Support for Everyone*. Available at www.gov.uk/government/uploads/system/uploads/attachment.data/file/215107/dh.133105.pdf, accessed on 2 October 2013.

Kubler-Ross, E. (1969) *On Death and Dying*. London: Taverstock.

MacLeod, R. (2007) 'Total pain – physical, psychological and spiritual.' *Goodfellow Symposium*. Available at www.fmhs.auckland.ac.nz/soph/centres/goodfellow/-docs/total_pain_handout.pdf, accessed on 17 June 2013.

Mayne, M. (1998) *Pray, Love, Remember*. London: Darton, Longman & Todd.

Monroe, B. (2008) Saunders, Cicely. *Oxford Dictionary of National Biography*. Oxford: Oxford University Press. Available at www.oxforddnd.com, accessed on 1 October 2008.

Monroe, B. and Oliviere, D. (2003) *Patient Participation in Pallitive Care – A Voice for the Voiceless.* Oxford: Oxford University Press.

Mount, B. (2003) 'The existential moment.' *Palliative & Supportive Care 1, 2,* 207.

Saunders, C. (1988) *St Christopher's in Celebration: 21 Years as Britain's First Modern Hospice.* London: Hodder & Stoughton.

Speck, P. (ed.) (2006) *Teamwork in Palliative Care: Fulfilling or Frustrating?* Oxford: Oxford University Press.

Twycross, R.G. (1974) 'Clinical experience with diamorphine in advanced malignant disease.' *International Journal of Clinical Pharmacology 9,* 184–198.

Weil, S. (1951) *Waiting for God: Reflections on the Right Use of Schools Studies.* Oakville, ON: Capricorn Books.

Chapter 3

Strategic and Current Challenges

Introduction

We now take a brief look at contemporary strategic imperatives and current challenges, specifically for hospices, but also for end of life care in general.

The following headings are used in order to address key areas:

- Background

- What is a strategic imperative?

- The conflict of need, demand and resource

- Excluded and vulnerable groups

- Changes in demographics

- Funding

- Case study

- Final thoughts.

The chapter will also highlight current publications by leading national bodies and examine the need for occupations such as the arts therapies and other allied health professions to mould their professional competences in order to fit within the current new directions for health and social care, as well as adhering and responding to both user and organisational requirements. The chapter will end with a story which links to the some of the main points raised.

Background

Why should you, as an artist or therapist, be aware of, or think seriously about, the strategic challenges that are facing the organisation for which you work or are interested in working with? When we train for any health care profession, we will be taught a range of skills and models, and possibly have the opportunity to practise these as part of a work-based placement. My experience has shown that there is often a tension between what we are taught to practise and how these things work in reality. More often than not, this can cause difficulty. It is very important that educational establishments keep up to date with changes that occur in the external field, but often this will not be the case (Hartley 2008). Therefore, the responsibility to learn and keep up to date with current changes in the health and social care sector will lie with the artists or therapists themselves.

Each organisation will have a current strategy, which will normally be set over a number of years, usually three to five. Outlined in this document will be the key points or areas that the organisation is wanting or needing to respond to over a period of time. It will be useful for you to have a look at this and identify any areas with which your particular line of work might engage effectively. It will be useful also to think how you might work to achieve some of the aims in partnership with others.

An example at St Christopher's is how changing attitudes about death and dying and the work that the hospice does has been part of our strategy for the last ten years or so. It is clear that the arts and the arts therapies have played a large role in enabling us to achieve much in this area, together with other professional groups and partnerships. Care of older people and changing people's experiences of coming to the end of life in a care home has also been a major strategic imperative. The hospice artists have supported a programme to enable this to happen through running short-term group projects and teaching sessions in care homes across South East London. This has been offered alongside a comprehensive nurse education package run by a specific care home team based at the hospice.

To be aware of organisational strategy is therefore not unimportant. If your need or aim is to offer only intensive one to one work to the users of an end of life care organisation, it is unlikely that such a service will have been identified as important for that client population. Reading and understanding the current organisational strategy will help you to place your work within a more necessary and useful framework as well as enabling you to appreciate the current essential needs of the organisation, the wider health and social care sector and, more important, the people who utilise its services.

We are already aware of the reasons behind Cicely Saunders' vision for a place where people's dying could be treated as a normal event and be well managed, and the impetus which resulted in the building of St Christopher's Hospice, London is clear and well documented. Even though there are now almost 300 hospices within the UK and end of life care initiatives in over 115 countries worldwide, considerable challenges still remain around the delivery and execution of good end of life care. Times change and the ways that people die also change. For example, dying in South East London in the 21st century provides issues and challenges that will be distinctly different than they were 45 years ago. In the 1960s it is likely that many parts of South East London were culturally and demographically very different and the changes in many communities and neighbourhoods across the world within the last 50 years have been vast. Today, for example, within the South East London catchment area of St Christopher's, the population is around 1.5 million people. The influx of new and diverse groups and cultures from across the world have brought with them different ways of life, together with different religious beliefs and practices (Scott *et* al. 2003). Parts of South East London also include communities which sit in the top quartile of poverty within the UK. These facts are important to know because they will *challenge* the delivery of existing health and social care models, provide pressure points and catalysts for change, and hopefully guide practice and help to formulate new ideas.

Every hospice or end of life care institution will serve a unique community of people, and because of this will need to develop and offer services in different ways from each other. When employed to work in a hospice as an artist or a therapist, it will be important that you know the community within which you are working as well as possible. This will, and should, have an impact on the kind of service that you offer. This knowledge will enable you to mould it and shape your work based on the needs of that community as they come to die.

What is a strategic imperative?

As already mentioned, most health and social care organisations will have a strategic plan which is written down. This strategic plan will set out the imperatives and priorities that the organisation sees as key for the foreseeable future, normally two to three years and sometimes as long as five years or more. In times of great societal change, it is likely that strategic plans will be shorter rather than longer, in order to give the opportunity to necessarily change them more frequently.

At the present time, for example, the strategic plan of a hospice might include the priority around providing end of life care education for generalist professions, growing the volunteer workforce through active recruitment and training, or growing in size due to joining up with other community providers and similar organisations to achieve a sense of scale.

Strategy is described as 'the direction and scope of an organisation over the long term, which achieves advantage in a changing environment through its configuration of resources and competences with the aim of fulfilling stakeholder expectations' (Johnson, Scholes and Whittington 2005, p.9). There are four key points to this description:

1. Direction and scope

2. Changing environment

3. Resources and competences

4. Stakeholder expectations.

Using hospice and end of life care services as an example, I would now like to examine each of the areas, albeit briefly, within the current health and social care climate.

1. Direction and scope

The direction and scope of an organisation will depend on many factors, including social, political and economic issues. For example, the main business of any hospice or end of life care service is, of course, dying. With some diseases, such as cancer, identifying the point when someone's illness becomes terminal has in the past been relatively straightforward. However, developments and trends in medicine with the emergence of new treatments provide challenges as people begin to live longer and require more extended care and support. The challenges of providing care for those people with long-term degenerative diseases and a range of neurological conditions also present some problems. As identifying 'dying' and the point of appropriate referral to an end of life care service becomes more complicated, the direction and scope of organisations providing services may need to change. Accepting referrals into services when patients are at an earlier stage in their illness or dying might prove a necessity for organisations in the future. As people live longer, the issue of 'survivorship' is something which is being addressed on a national scale by government and health and social care agencies. Living longer with dying and as people's illnesses become more chronic rather than terminal forces the provision of services to those who 'survive' into the market place. We would all think that people living longer can only be a good thing. However, there are dangers to consider. We must endeavour not to return to a time when death is seen as a failure and surviving is seen as the single successful goal. People will still die; the challenge for any organisation will continue to be how to care for people with a range of different illnesses along an ever changing continuum between diagnosis and death.

2. Changing environment

We live during a time of unprecedented change. A world-wide recession impacts on the lives that we live and on the work that we do. This financial pressure provides one of the biggest trials in living memory for the funding of both current and future health and social care provision across the world. At a time of global change comes difficulty, complexity and the need for precise decisions; however, there is also the potential and possibility for industries and services to transform themselves. As statutory funding bodies take time to review their systems and procedures, health and social care services can become more pressurised. Charities and not-for-profit organisations also find themselves struggling due to the general public having less money to give away to 'good causes'. Less money means that we all will have to experience different ways of living, maybe eating different kinds of food and wearing different kinds of clothes and changing our demands on, and expectations of, daily life. It goes without saying that a lack of money when we become ill will colour any experiences of illness, and also a lack of money when we come to die will colour our own experience of dying and also the experiences of our families and friends.

3. Resources and competences

Lack of funding can have a devastating effect on the resources that are available for people when they come to die. Hospices and end of life care services have been set up on the basis that people need more than general medical or nursing care as they come to the end of their life. As already mentioned in the previous chapter, the psychological, social and spiritual needs of those dying and their family members are also central to Saunders' model of holistic care. This means that good, effective end of life care is not a cheap option. However, during times of challenge, we all need to take an intelligent look at what we do and how we do it. This, of course, does not necessarily mean that quality care needs to be watered down. We are all probably guilty of not working to full capacity all of the time. The challenge is for us to look at what we do, and first of all ask if it is relevant to current need. The second thing we need to examine is whether we might change something of our practice to fit in with the changing needs of a shifting society. An example of this might be that as a therapist you have been taught to practise in a certain way. It might be that you will require to see people in a specially designed room. Your model might include seeing people at regular specific times for specific lengths of time. You might also be told that for your particular therapeutic model to work, you will need to see them over a lengthy period of time. With regard to fitting in this type of practice into end of life care we can sensibly observe that there may be problems.

1. Most end of life care in the UK is provided at home. Most hospices, for example, will only see about a quarter of the patient population within the hospice building at any one time. Needing to see people within a specifically designed room already prevents the three quarters of patients who will never visit the hospice building from benefitting from what you do.

2. Many people coming to the end of their life live most of their days not knowing what is going to happen next. On the whole, people's illnesses can change rapidly and regularly. They might find themselves needing to see medical or nursing practitioners at short notice in order to sort out specific problems. They may also find themselves admitted to hospital quickly and on multiple occasions, if their care is not co-ordinated speedily and effectively. Living their lives in

this way will make it impossible for many people to arrange appointments in advance. If your practice requires that you see the person in the same place at the same time every week, it will be impossible for many patients to benefit.

3. Many dying people will be under the care of a hospice or end of life care unit for a period of weeks or months. Regular on-going therapeutic work is therefore, in many circumstances, impossible to achieve. If your model of practice relies on people making long-term commitments and relationships, it will not fit the trajectory of most people's illnesses.

4. Stakeholder expectations

We can see that all of the points raised above are important. They are important because we can begin to understand that many of the needs of key stakeholders in end of life care might be conflicting to the practice of some professions. Here, we see a significant tension. It is therefore vital that our 'craft', as mentioned in Chapter 2, can be useful, not only to the users of end of life care services, but also to the organisations that provide their care, those who fund their care, and those that are responsible for policy and decision making regarding what that care should look like and how it might be provided. Key stakeholders in end of life care will include the following:

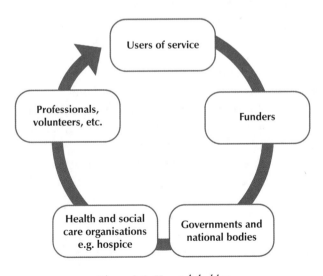

Figure 3.1: Key stakeholders

The conflict of need, demand and resource

In theory, all stakeholder groups should work effectively together in order to provide good quality, cost effective, useful care. In reality, there are normally many factors which interrupt the necessary flow for things to work successfully for the benefit of everyone involved. One example might be that training institutions might not be aware of new pressures or stresses facing health and social care organisations. As a result of this, they may miss the opportunity to change the nature of what they train professionals to do in the workplace. Changing the nature of what professionals do as part of their day to day job will be about constantly honing and refining the competences people need in order to work effectively. Equally, organisations which have provided good models of care over long periods of time may overlook the need to change their portfolio of services in order to better meet the changing needs of their user population. An example of this might be a hospice which fails to notice the changing landscape of death and dying. Failing to notice, for example, the growing need for care homes to provide better end of life care, or the need to 'skill-up' generalist professionals who provide most of the actual hands-on care within hospitals or within the home, could lead to the hospice becoming at best of limited use, or at worst irrelevant. It could also be that users of services demand a package of care which funders are unwilling to support and organisations unable to provide. Just because a large proportion of service users demand regular input from an aromatherapist, for example, will not mean that this is possible. It might be that many aromatherapy training programmes do not include sections on how to work with people who are dying so practitioners are inexperienced, or that funders cannot see the benefit of investing in a service which is unproven and they do not understand.

As mentioned earlier, if you are working for a hospice or end of life care organisation, or are applying for a position to work in one, it would be well worth your time to ask for a copy of their current strategic plan. The reason for this is that you may be able to better form your skill and craft appropriately in order to prove that you can address the demands of as many stakeholders as possible. You can also highlight that you have the necessary competences, and that your professional discipline has the relevant capacity, to be of use and to do what is needed in a cost effective and knowledgeable way.

Excluded and vulnerable groups

Many of us live as part of increasingly diverse communities. Indeed, some of us will belong to what are classified to be minority groups. As our society changes and develops, there is a danger that more and more people will experience exclusion or vulnerability. Many of these excluded or vulnerable groups can be listed as follows:

- black and minority ethnic groups
- those living in deprived areas
- people with mental health problems
- people with disabilities
- refugees and asylum seekers
- travellers
- prisoners
- the homeless
- drug and alcohol misusers
- carers
- those living with the 'wrong disease'.

Other people who are excluded or vulnerable might not be so noticeable, such as people who live alone with no family or friends to support them; those who are housebound because of their disease; the elderly who cannot get the care and support that they need; or a young carer of 15 who lives alone with her mother who has a rapidly advancing terminal cancer. All of these people, and others, present our society with dilemmas and challenges which might at times seem easier to put aside for another day. An important question for anyone intending to work in end of life care might be how does the professional discipline that you practise respond to the needs of excluded or vulnerable groups? This question is not about the benefits of what you can do to help these people, although this will be important to articulate. The question may be more about access, as unless you can actually get to these people, or find a way for them to get to you, hypothesising about the usefulness of art therapy or of hypnotherapy, for example, will be a futile exercise.

Changes in demographics

Many of us will be aware that the demographics of many communities are changing. For example, an ageing population means that by 2030, a higher percentage of all deaths will be of people over the age of 65, and around 40–50 per cent of all deaths will be of people over the age of 85 (Calanzani, Higginson and Gomes 2013). The increasing pressure to provide adequate care for older people will continue to be a key stressor for all health and social care providers in the years to come. Many of us will die in care homes, and due to living longer, it is probable that we will die from multiple, chronic illnesses, which may well include cancer and dementia. Focussing on finding solutions to such problems is becoming increasingly important. Many hospices and end of life care institutions are examining ways of establishing and developing good quality end of life care within care and residential homes. It is common in many major world cities that care within the majority of care homes is not quite as good as it should be. It is likely that when someone comes to die in a care home that many of the health and social care staff who work there will not feel confident and competent enough to support such residents who are actively dying. The result of this is that many older, dying people are taken to accident and emergency units by ambulance and then either die there, or are admitted to die on an inpatient ward in the local hospital. Equipping care home staff with the skills needed to care for an older, dying person within the bed that they have lived in for a number of years with those whom they know and trust around them is obviously paramount. Not only is admission into hospital via accident and emergency units expensive, it is also traumatic for the older person who will probably die within a stressful and unfamiliar environment. Training for care and residential home staff is therefore of the utmost importance in order to avoid such unnecessary admissions into hospital. In the UK, the development of the Gold Standards Framework (GSF), a training and recognition tool for care and residential home staff, is beginning to impact on this issue. Good care and good deaths in care and residential homes are not just, however, about getting nursing right. Helping care home residents to live until they die and to remain social beings is equally important. Your skill as a practitioner might be well-utilised by running groups for care home residents or teaching care and residential home staff or volunteers simple skills around 'life-story' work, or what is needed to work with residents in order to develop and sustain healthy and active relationships as they come to die.

Funding

Some people reading this book will belong to the many professions or groups that sit on the 'periphery' of end of life care such as artists, therapists, volunteers and others. All of the work we do has its price and in many cases the major issue will be about finding and retaining the right levels of funding in order to provide useful functions and services. It will be important therefore, that we persuade the right individuals and groups of people of our worth and use to those who might benefit from what we offer. In all financial climates, locating financial support and proving the worth of what we do will be key to acceptance and conviction. It is unlikely that lines of work other than medicine, nursing and the more established of allied health professions such as physiotherapy will be funded from statutory sources. This is helpful to know as wasting energy can be avoided by trying to convince the wrong people of the worth and value of what you do.

One major question for end of life care in the current climate is what should society pay for? We know that many hospice and end of life care units are registered charities, and on the whole, bring in the majority of their funding from local communities through a range of fundraising initiatives. Other charitable income might come from specific trusts and bodies which are set up to fund and develop specific areas of work.

Knowing that it is unlikely that the arts or therapy services within hospices will not be funded by statutory funding bodies, the energy expounded fighting for statutory funding for such activities might be better used in other ways, such as identifying appropriate trusts and other private funding bodies whose aims and objectives might include supporting the use of the arts or therapies in such settings. Funding applications in order to use the arts or different therapies will differ in size, from supporting the salary of a part or full-time artist to backing a short four to six week arts or therapy project. However small or large the application, it is important to focus on a number of key areas.

What follows is a simple guide in order to help put together a funding application for a small arts or therapy project.

Table 3.1: Sample funding application

1. *At the beginning of the proposal, include a title. Make sure this is clear and concise. It is important to also include here who will be responsible for overseeing the project.*
TITLE
Changing attitudes towards death and dying – a proposal to bring different community groups together with dying and elderly people in order to promote healthier attitudes
PROJECT LEAD
Art therapist
2. *The second part of the proposal should include a concise background. This should provide some information on how the arts have been used as part of hospice services in the past, or how the arts have successfully been used within hospices generally and how they have been proven to be useful within health promotion. It is important to include any references to successful evaluation and research that has been done.*
BACKGROUND
• Evidence and experience shows that people's relationship with the arts is heightened during illness. (How to format a simple funding proposal.)   • Over the past two years, using the arts has proved successful within the hospice and has enabled patients of all ages to have new experiences of themselves when they come to the end of their life. These experiences have enabled people to gain a deeper understanding of and clearer meaning in their own life, have provided a focus for the development of healthy relationships, and a means of enhancing and strengthening a sense of community.   • Due to a previous grant two years ago, we introduced the arts into the hospice day centre. Through offering a range of creative arts groups, we were able to create arrange of artwork which was recently exhibited to high acclaim at a number of prestigious art venues within our local community. As a result of these exhibitions, people's attitudes have been changed towards death and dying. This project will take the next step in engaging different community groups with dying and elderly people through the arts.
3. *The next section could include some information of how the money you are requesting will help the hospice to build on what it has learned from its past successes.*

BUILDING ON SUCCESS

- The hospice has developed and implemented a range of creative arts possibilities for patients and their carers as part of the day centre. During the past two years, due to the success of our existing arts project, our artist has also managed to work with a number of patients on our inpatient ward. Many of these patients, during the final days of their lives, have created art products which have been given to their loved ones as a keepsake.

- We plan to build on our successful programme, inviting community groups into the hospice building and also into a number of care homes within the local area.

- This additional funding would allow us to use the arts with people who would not otherwise have access to such a life-enriching experience within the places where they are living and dying and to bring them together with a range of other community groups in order to change attitudes and develop community responsibility.

- There is evidence to point to the increasing isolation of elderly people, due to geographical distance from family, or from limited family or other social support, and to a lack of provision of social and community support to these people in the last weeks of their life.

4. *It is now important to give a brief outline of how the project will be structured – explaining the length of the project, how the sessions will be offered and the plans for sustainability when the funding comes to an end.*

STRUCTURING THE PROJECT

- This project will take place over a 12-month period.

- We will build on and extend the creative arts opportunities available to patients within the hospice to groups of people coming to the end of their lives within care homes.

- Creative arts sessions will be delivered within the care home environment in order to support residents' psychological and social needs and to enable a deeper expression of meaning, identity and community.

- We plan to offer an introductory package of sessions to a group of care homes across the community which we serve. This would include two creative group sessions for residents, and an introductory creative group for care home staff while bringing into the care home community groups to engage with elderly residents through the arts. Our aim would be for the care homes to experience the benefit of such creative arts sessions for their residents and to examine further the possibilities of the continued funding of sessions from the care homes themselves.

- We plan to audit the project in order to identify how many care homes take up the possibility of buying further sessions for themselves and also to prove the efficacy of such work. We also plan to offer our findings to similar organisations in order to provide a template for future work.

cont.

5. *The final part of this simple funding proposal should include a breakdown of the budget. As well as including a breakdown of payment costs for the artist involved, it is important not to forget the costs of arts materials, and as the work is to take place within the local community, the costs of travel.*

BUDGET

- Cost per group session ****
- Material costs ****
- Travel costs ****

TOTAL **

If it is possible, include copies of artwork created in the past, as the majority of the time the reality of witnessing the work will be more important than the application itself. Also reference useful articles and research reports.

In all cases it will be important to build in, however simple, an evaluation tool as part of the project process. This could include basic qualitative questionnaires which could be filled in and analysed in order to identify successful key themes for future development. The evaluation tool could also include the analyses of audio or video recordings made of interviews during the process with key participants. Audio and video recordings could also be used as part of a future application process for further funding, as the recordings might provide valuable evidence of efficacy in themselves. It will also be important to keep quantitative data such as numbers of people who benefit from the project. Research and evaluation is covered in more depth in Chapter 11.

I am often approached by artists and therapists who want to use their skill and experience to work with hospice users. There are eight key steps to consider if you approach an organisation in this way:

1. Make sure that what you are offering can be of use both to the organisation and those who use it.

2. Make sure that you have the language in order to explain clearly what this use might be.

3. Research the evidence that proves that what you offer works and give examples of this.

4. Check that there is a 'gap' within the organisation's services which might be filled by what you can offer and that you are not replicating existing provision. Ask to see the organisation's

strategic plan beforehand. Make sure that what you offer is not 'too alternative' to be acceptable to the organisation's goals and mission.

5. Be clear on how much your service will cost.

6. Research possible sources of funding for a short pilot project, which should include an evaluation process. (Note that sometimes people approach organisations with their own funding. However, this does not necessarily mean that the proposal will work and will be a necessary fit to what is wanted and needed.)

7. Do not make claims about what you do that cannot be substantiated, and be realistic with what is possible.

8. Be open and flexible to mould and change your offer to fit with what is really needed.

Being drawn to work in a hospice or any other end of life care institution is only the beginning. It is important to understand both the environment that the organisation currently exists within, as well as understanding the sometimes very different needs and impetuses of the different stakeholders involved. In my experience, sometimes the educational and training establishments within which we learn to practise are the last group of stakeholders to realise that the needs of both the organisations who will employ future practitioners and those who use their services have changed and continue to do so. Persuading training programme leaders that this is the case can sometimes be complex and frustrating. Working on placement during training becomes increasingly important in order to change this pattern. Part of supervising students on placement might be instilling confidence in them and equipping and enabling them to return to their training institutions in order to paint a picture of what the world of health and social care really looks like. This is an important part of all health and social care providers' commitment and duty to the students who come to their organisations, and also to the training and education institutions which place them.

Case study: different stakeholder expectations

As already alluded to, there is sometimes a tension between our own professional discipline and what the key 'stakeholders' want and need and what we and our profession want to offer.

One hospice was keen to develop an arts programme for day care patients, but needed to prove that it worked before any funding could be applied for. In the past, art and craft groups had been offered as part of the hospice day care package by a small number of volunteers. The volunteers offered simple activities such as card making, making small mosaic objects and also watercolour painting. The lead day care nurse put together a simple questionnaire to gain some feedback from those who attended the groups and many patients voiced that they enjoyed these activities as it took their minds off their illnesses as well as gave them an enjoyable experience. Several patients also mentioned that it was fulfilling to give some of the work that they had made to family members or friends as a legacy. Acting on this feedback, the lead nurse had a desire to further establish the use of the arts and to gain some funding for a paid artist to come and work as part of the day care team. While she was looking for funding opportunities, she learned that in the nearby city, the local university offered a Master's programme in art therapy. She decided to approach the course leader to see if it was possible to learn more about the discipline that they taught. The tutor mentioned to her that it might be possible for a student to come to the hospice on a placement. It was common that students went on placement to various institutions, but normally when an art therapist worked there already, in order to model and supervise the work. However, the tutor said to the nurse that as she had a counselling qualification herself, and if she agreed to take on the supervision of the student, he would be able to send a student to the hospice. He also said that in addition to weekly supervision, the student would be expected to run a group and work with one or two patients on an individual basis. This sounded fine to the nurse, and she was pleased that the day care attendees would be able to benefit from art therapy with no cost to the hospice.

In order for the student to run a group in day care, the nurse needed to ask the volunteers to stop running their activities for a while. She was extremely surprised that the volunteers were very upset with this as they enjoyed running the groups and for a few of them it was the reason that they volunteered their time to the hospice. The volunteers also began to speak to the patients who then became upset on the volunteers' behalf, picking up on the term 'art therapy', stating that they did not need or want 'therapy' as there was nothing wrong with them. The nurse had not expected such a strong reaction from both patients and volunteers and continued to try hard to persuade them to co-operate and try out the new arrangement. She promised the volunteers that they would be able to help the student and that not very much would actually change.

The student eventually arrived on placement. This was the first time they had been to a hospice, so it was new territory to them. The model of art therapy that they were being taught and expected to practise was heavily based within psychodynamic theory. As a result of this, the student said that they required a private room in order to run a group and any individual sessions. This was difficult to arrange, as the day care centre was very open plan and normally groups took place alongside other day to day events.

It just so happened that all of this coincided with the 20th anniversary of the hospice. Celebrations were being planned for a major event in a few months' time which would include a large service in the city cathedral with which the hospice had strong links. The chief executive of the hospice was keen that some of the artwork created in day care should be exhibited during the service, in order to give funders and supporters of the hospice some concrete examples of what was offered to, and what was achieved by, patients and families.

We begin to see here that there are many different expectations around how the arts should be used and a major potential for conflict and misunderstanding.

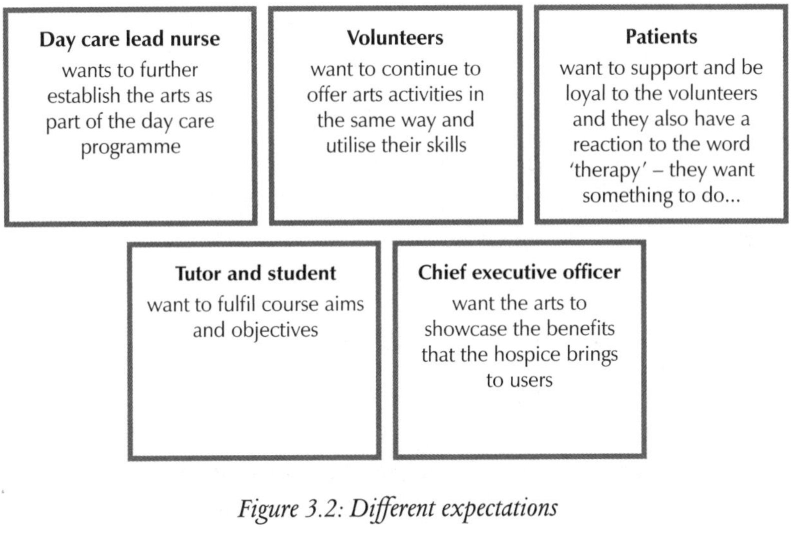

Day care lead nurse	**Volunteers**	**Patients**
wants to further establish the arts as part of the day care programme	want to continue to offer arts activities in the same way and utilise their skills	want to support and be loyal to the volunteers and they also have a reaction to the word 'therapy' – they want something to do...

Tutor and student	**Chief executive officer**
want to fulfil course aims and objectives	want the arts to showcase the benefits that the hospice brings to users

Figure 3.2: Different expectations

This figure provides a clear example of some the issues which arise when a range of different key people involved in a process do not have similar wants, needs or expectations. However, there was a good outcome to this story.

The student involved contacted an experienced art therapist who had worked in hospices for many years. The experienced art therapist worked in another hospice which was only a few miles away from the university where the student was studying, and following agreement with the tutor and the day care lead nurse, took on the weekly supervision of the student placement. This relationship became an important catalyst and began to help to bring together the key groups involved in a constructive way. The art therapist supervisor helped the student to find some referrals of individual patients who were not attending the hospice day care centre, but were either staying on the inpatient ward of the hospice or could come to the hospice as an outpatient. The supervisor also introduced the student to a well tried art therapy group work model. This particular model involved the student directing the patients through a range of specific ideas using the method of focussing them in each group work session to create artwork around key themes. The student also ran a separate session with the volunteers, which helped develop their understanding and gain their commitment to working in a different way. It is interesting to note that as the volunteers became more engaged and involved, so did the patients. One of the aims of the art group was that, with the patients' permission, the artwork would be exhibited as part of the hospice anniversary celebrations. The experienced art therapist provided the missing piece in order to enable the different stakeholders to come together in a cohesive way.

Art therapist
using their expertise and experience to join things together and to fill in 'gaps' in knowledge

---

Figure 3.3: The missing piece

This story highlights the importance of taking time to understand the different expectations of the key groups of people who are involved with a project. As the expectations may be different, it will be essential to take time to comprehend the motivation and needs of each group in order for the potential and possibility for a more cohesive result to be practised and realised.

Final thoughts

We must never fool ourselves into thinking that those people coming to the end of their lives can always benefit from what we have to offer them. In reality, it is much more complex than this. We need to take an interest in, and understand, the broader health and social care environment in order to be able to remould and re-evaluate our craft and skills to be relevant and useful. In some cases, we may need to do this on a regular basis.

I have known many accomplished musicians and artists, who when trained as arts therapists have somehow forgotten the importance of the musical and artistic in their work in favour of various therapeutic models and professionalised languages. What I mean by this is that the quality and value of the artwork often takes second place to what occurs in the relationship between the therapist and the client. In contrast, it has always been clear to me that the art is the therapy. The word 'therapy' should not just be used after the word 'arts' to give us as practitioners a sense of importance and acceptance within the health and social care professional framework. The arts are unique, and it is this uniqueness which brings to organisations and those who use them both something fresh and new and also a dynamic way of meeting some internal and external strategic drivers. It is straightforward to see that art exhibited and performed within health care settings can bring a sense of vitality and purpose to the everyday life of the institution. When the work is created by those people who use health and social care services, it can give reasons to stop and look or to learn and listen, as well as give a sense of community, belonging and purpose (Hartley and Payne 2008).

Understanding what drives the present and future needs of people coming to the end of their lives is crucial. It is clear that being able to change the lives and deaths of one or two individuals does not warrant the need for whole professional groups to be developed and utilised. Being committed and able to change the lives and deaths of whole communities of people needs to sit at the core of any future health and social care profession. If we can achieve this, then we might well be seen as a useful part of the brave new, broader world of patient-led health and social care driven by a complex mix of varied user need and limited financial and professional resources (Hartley 2008).

References

Calanzani, N., Higginson, I. J. and Gomes, B. (2013) *Current and Future Needs for Hospice Care: An Evidence-based Report. Help the Hospices Commission into the Future of Hospice Care.* London: Help the Hospices.

Hartley, N. (2008) 'The arts in health and social care –is music therapy fit for purpose?' *British Journal of Music Therapy 22*, 2, 88–96.

Hartley, N. and Payne, M. (2008) *The Creative Arts in Palliative Care.* London and Philadelphia, PA: Jessica Kingsley Publishers.

Johnson, G. Scholes, K. and Whittington, R. (2005) *Exploring Corporate Strategy: Texts and Cases.* 7th edition. Harlow: Prentice Hall Financial Times.

Scott, T., Mannion, R., Davies, H.T.O., Marshall, M.N. (2003) 'Implementing culture change in health care: theory and practice.' *International Journal of Quality Health Care 15*, 2, 111–118.

PART 2

Teamwork, Communication and Working in Different Contexts

Chapter 4

Working as Part of a Multi-disciplinary Team

Tamsin Dives and Nigel Hartley

Introduction

There has been much written about the benefits of the arts and variety of other therapies for those coming to the end of their life (Hartley and Payne 2008). However, how the arts and some therapies fit into a multi-disciplinary team approach has rarely been addressed. Many published case studies of the arts in palliative care showcase their efficacy when used with people facing the end of life, facilitated by the artist as an individual practitioner. Nevertheless, at the core of multi-disciplinary team work lie the benefits of working as a 'complete team', with success and failure being owned by the team as opposed to any individual practitioner.

With regard to the impact of the arts in end of life care, the lack of reference as to how this is achieved in collaboration with other professions as part of a co-ordinated care plan is possibly due to the need for a stronger integration of the profession into the culture of multi-disciplinary working. This is true because use of the arts within the area of palliative care is still very much in its infancy.

Despite the work of a handful of pioneers over the past 20 years, substantial posts for artists in hospices remain rare, and where posts do exist, they consist of sporadic, part-time work. Part-time hours make it difficult for the artist to experience the full benefits of working as part of a multi-disciplinary team as it is often the case that the artist does not work on a day when the team meetings are held. Therefore, the artist will not have adequate opportunities to feed back about their involvement within a patient's care or to learn from other professionals in the team in any formal way. It is also true that the growth in the number of postgraduate arts and arts therapies students using hospices as placement organisations does not appear to offer a solution to the problem. Most training courses in the UK, indeed across the world, offer short-term placements of one or two days a week in different institutions. Again, the student is rarely able to attend multi-disciplinary meetings due to their sporadic attendance in the workplace. In addition, they get little opportunity to learn about organisational culture and end of life care treatment models. Until the academic institutions which offer training for artists can address this through redeveloping education programmes, the cycle will continue.

It will not be unusual, therefore, in an organisation which may have employed an artist for a number of years, to come across key members of the multi-disciplinary team who know little about what the artist can offer to patients and their families.

St Christopher's Group, which comprise both St Christopher's Hospice and Harris HospisCare with St Christopher's, although one of the largest in the UK with a workforce of around 300 paid staff, is typical in terms of the different groups of professionals it employs which make up the multi-disciplinary team. It is vital that teams learn how to share, and experience sharing, their knowledge, skills and values. Peter Speck (2006) lists some of the important values of multi-disciplinary teamwork:

- the importance of working together to achieve the aim

- each team member deserves respect

- open and honest communication

- open access to information.

Living out these values on a day to day basis is not straightforward. It demands commitment from individual members of the team. Therefore, the inability to attend multi-disciplinary team meetings where these values will be practised and accomplished means that both the artist or the therapist, and their role, will struggle to be integrated fully, either into the team of professionals, or into the patient's care plan.

During this chapter, we hear from Tamsin who is an experienced professional musician and music therapist. She shares with us her experiences of working as part of a large multi-disciplinary team within St Christopher's Hospice. Some of her experiences mirror what has been mentioned earlier within this introduction, and after describing her background, she outlines her experiences under the following headings:

- The multi-disciplinary team

- Challenges of professional discourse: talking about what we do

- Record keeping

- Integrating into different teams

- Management structures

- The hospice community

- Students on placement.

Tamsin also includes a number of short case studies in order to illustrate the points which she raises and the chapter ends with my reflections and considerations.

Tamsin: my background

My name is Tamsin Dives and during my career of 25 years as a professional opera singer I often needed to engage myself in some work other than music. In the 1980s I became a volunteer with the Terence Higgins Trust. The HIV/AIDS pandemic shaped and dominated the lives of many of my peers, bringing with it fear, together with a lack of understanding. Many of my colleagues and friends contracted the virus and many died as a result of it. Later on as a young mother I was active in the local community of my children's school, interested in bringing different groups and cultures together through using art, performance and music. In my mid-forties, certain aspects of the music business began to disappoint me and I looked for a complete career change. I went back to college for a second time, originally having studied singing, this time I retrained as a music therapist. I remember attending a number of introduction to music therapy days, in order to decide on which training course I was most suited to. These days consisted of a range of presentations from different areas of music therapy work, and I remember that the ones which really struck me were in the areas of dementia and palliative care. My training to become a music therapist at the Guildhall School of Music and Drama was only a year long. At the time, this suited me well as my children were still at school. However, there was a lot to cover in one year and I found it extremely full-on. Having graduated, I set upon the difficult task of finding a job. I initially fell into the trap of agreeing to the bits and pieces of music therapy work which I was offered, ending up juggling many small jobs with different groups of people in a range of geographical locations. Eventually, I got a job working as a music therapist at St Christopher's three days a week and then I became part of a larger team of artists which worked in a variety of places and in a variety of ways on behalf of the hospice. As a performing musician who specialised in opera, I was used to being a team player. I had experienced that being a musician was all about partnership, working as part of a group of people with the same aims and goals in mind. In fact, in my experience, no one was offered work as a performing musician if they could not fit in with other players, and I discovered that personality and good communication skills were essential to a successful performance. The truth is that working as part of a complex team was not a new experience for me when I first worked in end of life care.

When I applied for the job at St Christopher's Hospice, the job description stated that much of the job entailed liaising with a range of different professionals, fitting into a variety of teams and building relationships with different professional groups. In fact, the ability to work within a team is not unique to working in end of life care, and is a prerequisite for most jobs in most organisations. Within health care particularly though, working successfully from a team perspective has proved to offer a more connected experience for the patient and has also given the potential to deliver services in a more cost effective way (Speck 2006).

It is not difficult for us to imagine the value and importance of working with other professionals in groups and teams when people's health and wellbeing are the major focus. Throughout our lives we join and leave many groups. Some of our group experiences will be positive and enabling, and at other times we might feel left out of the group and misunderstood. All of these experiences will stay with us and will influence our future experiences of being in a group; however, the more positive experiences can enable us to accrue the skills to communicate well, to interact with others and to belong.

Dame Cicely Saunders, the founder of the modern hospice movement, coined the phrase 'total pain', describing it as 'the division of a whole experience into physical, emotional, social and spiritual components' (Saunders and Sykes 1993, p.305). She advocated a quality of care that should be delivered by more than one person. A multi-disciplinary approach defines this, a working practice where each professional and each professional group can be as important as the other. It is argued that this way of thinking and acting together around the care of a dying person can assist them in maintaining their maximum potential right to the end of their lives.

The process of dying is multi-layered and palliative care draws on a broad spectrum of disciplines, knowledge, skills, experience and creative thought. For example, although pain and symptom management is a vital component in good end of life care, there are many aspects other than medicine supporting the dying process, and it is unlikely that all of the components can be delivered by one professional. As stated by the Department of Health in their publication *Valuing People* (2001), 'specialist services should be planned and delivered with the focus on the whole person ensuring a continuity of provision and appropriate partnership between agencies and professions' (p.75).

Team work, therefore, is an essential and integral part to good palliative care; in fact, it is central both to its provision and its success.

Barbara Monroe (2006, p.203) suggests that 'the necessity for and the utility of multi-disciplinary teams in palliative care has become an almost automatic assumption. The assumption stems from an understanding of the need to integrate and coordinate the multiple skills and complex knowledge base required to deliver the holistic care to which palliative care aspires.'

Working as part of the multi-disciplinary team at St Christopher's Hospice has obviously influenced my experience of being part of a large team of artists within the organisation. I aim to share with you my experiences in the following way:

- from my perspective as a trained music therapist

- through sharing the strengths to my working practice and also some of the issues and challenges that emerge

- through acknowledging the benefits that working in this way can bring to the patient and their family as well as to the team and to the organisation

- by considering how the artist needs to determine and negotiate a way of working together with a range of different health care professionals.

The multi-disciplinary team

I remember a quote from Robert Redford, who said that 'problems can become opportunities when the right people come together'. The multi-disciplinary team at St Christopher's is made up of many different professionals including nurses, doctors, physiotherapists, occupational therapists, a chaplain, as well as art therapists and social workers. An example of how the team looks is below, supporting patients and families across three contexts, the inpatient unit, the Anniversary/Caritas Centre (day and outpatients) and the community (people's own homes, care homes and social care).

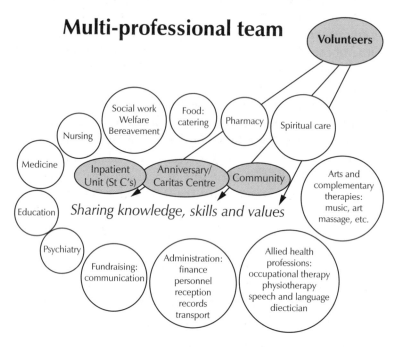

Figure 4.1: An example of the multi-disciplinary team at the St Christopher's Group, supporting the three contexts of the inpatient wards, day and outpatient services, and home care and other community venues

Some members of the multi-disciplinary team will be involved with a patient from when they are referred to the hospice until the time they die. For other professionals, it might be just one or two specific interventions as part of the patient's care. The multi-disciplinary team is designed to manage all aspects of care and when this works well, I have witnessed numerous benefits for the patient and their family members and carers, as well as for members of the multi-disciplinary team alike. A team can offer a broad combination of complementary crafts and skills. The range of the different kinds of professionals belonging to the team means that work can be carried out more effectively and with a more flexible approach. As a complete unit it is certainly able to address problems and turn them into opportunities. Through sharing skills and information the team is also able to broaden the impact of the care it offers. If conflict arises in the team I have discovered that it is not necessarily a bad thing and that it may well lead to solving problems in a more creative way, as different perspectives can often offer new and dynamic ways of viewing things (Crawford and Price 2003). Of course, a team approach can expose individual weaknesses, but it can also maximise the strengths that different professionals have, with the whole being greater than the sum of its parts.

In palliative care, I have observed that the patient and family are central to their own treatment. This suggests an active participation from the patient and their family members in the way that their care is managed (Orchard and Curran 2003). Patients benefit from this multi-disciplinary approach, and this offers them a greater sense of choice about their care at a time when they might not be experiencing any sense of control in any area of their lives.

With the internet at our fingertips, which can give us information in an instant, patients and their families are often more enlightened about their care and more knowledgeable about what might be available for them. This can be empowering for the patient and the family but can also make things more challenging for the professional (Oliviere 2006). Knowledge is not always a good thing, especially when much information on the internet can be conflicting and confusing. In my experience, there are also patients who insist that they do not want any information about their diagnosis and/or disease progression. This has to be respected and carefully managed from a whole multi-disciplinary team perspective.

Patient's needs and wishes may well change many times during the process of dying and I have learned that a team which includes many disciplines and viewpoints can only support this and be useful through good communication and sharing of information. There are sometimes occasions when a patient's needs and expectations are considerable, and other times when this is less so. In my experience good communication among the multi-disciplinary team members can help to support patients and their family members and friends by offering practical options and support in a timely manner.

The following story demonstrates how a multi-disciplinary team can address the complexities of death and dying for a particular patient and their family and also how music therapy can fit usefully into this.

Case study: 'V.' – addressing the whole family's needs through multi-disciplinary work

A woman dying with cancer was referred to the music therapist by the social worker. V. the patient, was married with a teenage daughter. She was anxious about the relationship between her daughter and her father (the patient's partner) and wanted the family to work through some of these issues with professional support, while she was still well enough to participate. We explained to V. and her partner that music therapy might offer the family a different kind of opportunity to meet and explore their relationships and some of their feelings together. I worked with the family for some months. It was extremely useful to be able to share and reflect on the work with my colleagues from within the multi-disciplinary team, which included the social worker, and to share with her how the work was progressing. In this instance the social worker, in particular, was able to let us know how music therapy was supporting the family as part of their life together within the home.

During our music sessions, the family explored their relationships through musical games and improvisation. The daughter began to see her father in a very different way. They were able to laugh together, tease each other and also explore painful feelings, which were sometimes released through the musical improvisations which we created together. Relationships changed and it seemed that they all found some new strength to face what was happening. It was also important for V. to see these developments before she died. Following her death, the daughter accessed support from the Candle Project, a child bereavement initiative based at St Christopher's, which offers group counselling and suport for children experiencing loss through death. The daughter was able to meet with teenagers who were also experiencing the death of a family member. The father also went on to seek support from one of the hospice welfare officers, who was able to help him sort out some debt problems. V's requirements changed throughout her illness and the team was also able to address these. As a team we supported the family and after V's death the care continued. Her husband still comes into the hospice for support by attending the Social Programme and the daughter is able to contact the child bereavement project when she needs to.

Challenges of professional discourse: talking about what we do

As already mentioned, there are many challenges to multi-disciplinary team working. Working in a palliative care environment can be difficult and I find that myself and my colleagues are sometimes confronted with issues which will resonate personally (Ramsay 2006). These issues can sometimes create tensions and I have found that we all need to challenge each other from time to time.

One of the major difficulties I have found is the need to develop an understanding of a wide range of different professional discourses and languages. We will all use and develop our own unique way of talking about the work that we do. The doctor will often talk about different types of medication and treatments, some of which I will find familiar and others will be new to me. Sometimes one nurse will use a different kind of language to another, even when they are both, in reality, attempting to describe the same thing. It is not always possible to gain a complete understanding of what other professionals are saying in a meeting, sometimes there is a chance to say 'could you explain this a little more?' or 'I don't understand what is being said.' This is not often appropriate in the meeting itself, but it is good to remember that it is always possible to speak with people, or to research and look things up after the meeting is over.

From another perspective, of course, we know that as artists it is equally important how we articulate the work we do into a format that makes sense as part of a care plan which is delivered by a number of different health care professionals. Why is it important that a person paints a picture, writes a poem or beats a drum in a certain way? We need to find ways of articulating answers to such questions in a way that is clear and uncomplicated.

My experience has shown that it can be an easy option for artists and arts therapists, when struggling to explain their work, to rely too heavily on psychotherapeutic or psychological theory. I have found that there can be a professional rivalry, especially among those professions who work within psychological or psychotherapeutic frameworks. We can sometimes try and set our work as artists within languages which lend themselves to both of these areas, the result of which can occasionally seem as if we are attempting to do the same job as the psychologist, counsellor or social worker. It is important that we struggle to articulate what the arts can bring to the table which is unique to them. This can include the possibilities for offering different structures and contexts, particularly when people are unable to articulate what is happening to them verbally. For instance, creating music together with the musician or music therapist offers the potential for an active, dynamic relationship in a way that many other professions do not focus on: the fact that the musician or music therapist and patient play together at the same time is unique to this profession. Also, with art or music, the product can act as proof of efficacy and this can offer a useful perspective for the multi-disciplinary team to take into consideration. I have discovered that taking and sharing artwork or playing recordings of music therapy sessions, as part of the multi-disciplinary team meeting, can unlock an awareness and a new understanding of the place of the arts within an effective care plan for patients. Words are not the only way to communicate.

Case study: the immediacy and intimacy of music

I played the piano and the patient sat beside me in his wheelchair. The pace of the music I improvised was very much aligned to the patient's breathing patterns. The music developed into a gentle waltz, with a clear three-beat structure. The patient began to vocalise (ba, ba) on the second and third beats of the bar. As the waltz developed I played louder and the patient's interjections became more rhythmic and confident.

Record keeping

My experience has taught me that careful and clear documentation is essential. Every arts session is recorded in the patient's multi-disciplinary notes. At St Christopher's, we use an electronic system (EPR), which I have needed to study and learn about in order to navigate and utilise it effectively. Other organisations use paper notes which are hand written. I try to keep my findings concise and simple, and some examples of this are given below:

> *Music Therapy – 1:1 session:* T. entered the room in a highly emotional state. He stated he did not want to talk but wanted to play the drums. He played chaotically and loudly. I joined him at the piano and after a while his playing became more ordered. As he left at the end of the session he said he'd felt 'listened to'.

Music Therapy – 1:1 session: Although C.'s motor control is severely reduced she can beat a drum and cymbal and we are able to improvise together. She seems encouraged by what she is able to achieve.

Music Therapy – 1:1 session: I noticed that W. was able to move in a much more relaxed manner after music therapy than before.

Members of the multi-disciplinary team can see, by reading the patient's notes, how many art or music sessions have taken place and how they are progressing. It is also a way of bringing the arts and music to the attention of all multi-disciplinary team members. I always look at the multi-disciplinary notes before working with a new patient. It is an opportunity to gain an idea of which professionals from the team are already working with the patient and why, and also to garner useful information about the patient before meeting them.

Integrating into different teams

It is true to say that many hospices will have more than one multi-disciplinary team. At the simplest level, there will be at least one team for the inpatient unit, one for the day centre, and another for the community. The larger the hospice, the more complex this might be for the artist or arts therapist who might be the only person to represent their particular professional group. In reality, at St Christopher's there are four inpatient wards, each with their own multi-disciplinary team meeting, as well as five community multi-disciplinary teams, and one multi-disciplinary team for the day care function, known as the Anniversary Centre. Each multi-disciplinary team meets at St Christopher's once a week. There might be up to 15 people in the meeting with one hour to discuss up to six patients. Therefore, time is precious and meetings need to be led and managed efficiently. I have learned not to say something just for the sake of it. This is the forum where you can represent yourself professionally alongside other professionals. However, everyone comes from a different discipline, describing and thinking about their work in different ways (Sutton 2008). Language and the way we use it is therefore vital if we and our work is to be fully understood. I have also discovered that this is not the place to be mysterious about the way we do our work.

Case study: structure

When recently discussing a patient with a physiotherapist I noticed we were able to use the same language about our work. The patient was wheelchair-bound and was working with the physiotherapist to regain the use of his legs and to strengthen the use of his arms. We talked together about ways to improve the patient's mobility. We realised 'structure' was a key word in the way we described our work with this particular gentleman. The physiotherapist used the parallel bars to support the patient as he began to walk again. She explained some of the coping skills and strategies she was offering to the patient and the physical support that was available to him. She spoke of rhythm. I suggested that the music we made together in our sessions equally offered him opportunities to initiate movement and I was able to explain that musical form and structure gave him support, improving his motor function and helping him to motivate and control his movements.

As an artist I find that I need to integrate into these different multi-disciplinary teams at different times, and, as I have mentioned before, I cannot underestimate the common problem that artists regularly face, due to the part-time nature of their work, of not being able to attend team meetings.

Management structures

I am reminded of something that Henry Ford once said, that 'coming together is a beginning, keeping together a process, working together a success'. The arts within a health care organisation can often have a very visible profile. Working as a musician or as a music therapist, your work can often be heard as music creeps out of rooms and down the corridors. Working as an artist or arts therapist, art created together with patients, carers, staff and volunteers might be displayed on the walls of the building. I have found that performances and exhibitions of work can be very important in showing the efficacy of both music and the arts, and can also be a useful part of the process for patients and families who have been involved in the arts projects.

In my current role, I am line-managed by someone who used to work as an arts therapist. I am also fortunate enough to work together with a large team of artists and arts therapists. However, this has not always been the case when I have worked in other institutions. With regard to working in hospices, it is likely that a music or arts therapist, or other kind of artist, will be the sole professional providing such a service, and will also usually work part time. In this case, it is common that an artist will be managed by a nursing or social work lead, or possibly the chaplain or psychologist or someone who manages the day care services. I have come to realise that who we are managed by can be extremely important. It is likely that the person managing us will have their own relationship with music and the arts, and the nature of this relationship can be both powerful and very influential. We also know that each one of us who works as an artist or arts therapist is also influenced by music and the arts within our own lives, and it is very important that we are aware of this influence in order to use music and the arts with people effectively when they are sick and vulnerable.

Case study: a nurse manager's emotional issues

A music therapist, who is managed by a nurse manager in the hospice where she works, told me that the nurse was worried about how music might have too powerful an effect on people as they approach the end of their lives. The nurse was concerned that music was evoking powerful feelings that overwhelmed patients and made them unable to cope. A while later, during conversation with the nurse, it transpired that she used to enjoy singing in the church choir. However, since the death of her mother a couple of years earlier, she had stopped singing, as she found it too distressing. It is likely that such experiences will colour our relationships with music and the arts, and this in turn can influence us in many different ways.

Being line-managed by someone who has previously worked as an artist, although hugely beneficial, can also have its drawbacks. Sometimes, I have found that I do not always feel free to try things out from my own perspective, being influenced by someone who has much more experience of working in the field. However, I also know and value the creative insight and energy that comes from both being managed by an artist, and also working alongside a number of different artists. At St Christopher's our on-site open group work programme is structured into eight-week blocks. This means that arts groups are led by a different member of the team every eight weeks and we run groups in the community and in care homes on the same basis. If you are working alone as an artist in an organisation, I find that when working with groups, having a definitive beginning and ending to a project can be extremely useful. By the very nature of hospices, the group membership changes quickly, and changing the focus of a group can be beneficial when constantly needing to welcome in new people. At St Christopher's, we offer people a variety of mediums and approaches as part of their experiences. We meet every two weeks as a team and alternate between a meeting where we plan what needs to be done and another when we can bring problems to share. It is a useful forum in which to reflect and share work processes and a place where we can describe our work and share a common understanding.

As artists, I find that we are constantly working in different contexts and we are always negotiating different territories. The sociologist Sennett argues that although there are great strengths to multi-disciplinary working there can be problems as different professional groups can hold on fiercely to their expertise, not wishing to share their knowledge. We face expectations from patients, staff, the organisation and ourselves, and as we move through these various territories we are constantly negotiating the meaning and purpose of our work. It is true that every individual member of the multi-disciplinary team has their own protocol, a way of dealing with things, and possibly a need to protect their own sphere of influence and territory.

I have certainly felt often that some health care professionals are territorial about their patch. An example of this is when, as a music therapist, I play and sing music on the wards. A member of staff might say – 'don't play something sad', 'make sure it's happy', 'there's no point in playing to them they're too ill'.

All of this impacts on how I can practise my work as a music therapist. I think that as artists, we can represent for people the possibility of doing something new in a different way. At times, this newness and difference can be challenging and difficult for our colleagues. If a boundary is a guarded place, the border, the interface, can become an active edge, a place of tension.

Case study: 'Moon River'

I remember singing 'Moon River' to a patient on the wards. A nurse took me aside afterwards saying that she felt the song was not appropriate. Quoting 'wherever you're going, I'm going your way', she worried that the patient might feel this was about his impending death and that we wouldn't be 'going his way'. This was a 'difficult' moment for me but offered us a chance to share some ideas about my work and her fears about what I was doing. This opportunity to talk about our approaches was invaluable.

It is important to realise that there can also be a hierarchy within the multi-disciplinary team which needs to be considered. This is to be expected, and in many circumstances, is entirely right. For the most part, we have to realise and understand that the medical consultant, nurse and social worker are going to be very important figures to most patients and their families. When someone is in great physical pain, my experience has shown that, for the patient, spending some time with the specialist nurse or medical consultant is far more important than spending time with the artist or arts therapist. I have discovered that it is best to acknowledge this from a place of understanding and humility and attempt to always see it from the patient's perspective. This does not mean to say, however, that the arts are never important or crucial to patients and their families, but I feel that this needs to be understood within the context of the lived experience.

Our work is not always protected by a closed door. We need confidence, and need other members of the multi-disciplinary team to also have some confidence, in our own knowledge and abilities as professional artists. This confidence and trust should help others to understand that we are working as professionals in an informed and responsible manner, even when the public nature of our work might appear otherwise to other people. To do this, it has become clear to me that we need to be managed well.

The hospice community

As the arts have developed and grown over the years at St Christopher's, I see that we are all becoming more flexible and imaginative about how we do things, and I guess that this comes with experience. However, whether you belong to a team of artists, or are a lone practitioner working part time among a broad group of different health care professionals, this does takes time. The trust and freedom my manager gives us about the way we work does encourage this more creative and flexible approach. Our work is defined by patients' needs and this is lived out as we come together with the rest of the multi-disciplinary team to meet the needs of the 'whole' patient.

I find that I am often doing things I never imagined I would, working in mediums other than music – spoken word and poetry, film making, puppetry – and I find this both refreshing and stimulating. Sometimes, you may find yourself needing to defend your work, your particular art form, to the point where you might lose all sense of creativity. Working as an artist, we must strive to keep our creativity central to our workplace experience, to use it to gently challenge and provoke as well as to motivate and innovate.

Occasionally, I do find that the variety of things that I and my arts team colleagues offer can seem somewhat confusing to other people. For example, alongside more conventional one to one and group music therapy, I play the piano in the hospice public spaces, run a community choir, perform to certain groups, put up pictures; and I am always moving chairs! The arts can transform public places quickly, changing exhibitions, displaying different kinds of work. We must not underestimate how this has an immediate effect for other people within the workplace (Stokes 1994). As artists we are an important part of both the physical and the emotional environment within the organisation which has the potential to impact all of those who use it.

St Christopher's Hospice is a community and as such all life is present. There is a large central space where patients and visitors gather known as the Anniversary Centre. Patients access whatever they wish and might well be sitting alongside someone who has just popped in from the local community to have a coffee. We have a café area with good food, internet access, places to sit and relax and beautiful gardens. Members of the local community are welcomed in. For example, we have a regular professional concert series which the public pay to attend. There is live music each Sunday while patients, families, friends and visitors have lunch together. All of the artwork that is displayed on the walls at St Christopher's has been created by patients and other users of the building, including staff and volunteers. In this way, the arts, as well as offering possibilities for patients and carers, can act as on-going refreshment for our fellow members of the multi-disciplinary team. The changing exhibitions are a way of 'marking' and celebrating this diverse and dynamic community.

Students on placement

A variety of health care students as part of their training are commonly on placement within most hospices. At St Christopher's, we also have students from various arts therapies and arts training programmes who come and spend time with us as part of their education. Acting as a placement supervisor is an option for most hospice staff or for the artists and arts therapist who work there. On a positive note, a student can add some human resource to an often limited arts service and can be supervised by an artist who is experienced in practising within this particular area. From another perspective, students can be time consuming within an already stretched timetable, and if they do not work well, can create problems across the whole multi-disciplinary team. In order for placements to work well and if they are going to be of any value, the students need to be present for reasonable lengths of time. Two or three days a week for around six months works well, as it takes time to get to grips with working in end of life care and the impact it has. I have also found that it works best if a student begins to work with day and outpatients, moving on to inpatients and visiting people within their own homes later in the placement. However, it is important that students get a varied experience across the whole spectrum of end of life contexts. After all, most people receive most of their care at home, and the student needs to gain experience of providing this if they are to become useful practitioners for the future.

In terms of my own training I did not realise how important it was going to be to articulate, clearly and precisely, my work to other professionals, and this is something I continue to improve and develop. Moving from being a student to being a paid professional, I have found that I need to let go of a lot of what I was trained to do. For example, most of my training taught me to work within the confines of a strict therapeutic frame and clear boundaries but, in reality, this is rarely the case, and often the patient wants family members or friends to join in. Of course, some of my work is behind a closed door for an agreed number of weeks, but this is infrequent.

Case study: 'B.' and his family

I went to work with B. on the inpatient ward. In conversation we had discussed song writing and I took to the session a keyboard, recording device, paper, and a selection of songs B. had mentioned as particularly meaningful to him. When I got to the room, his wife and teenage daughter were sitting with him. He was not well enough to engage in song writing but asked if I would sing to him. The three sat, holding hands, B. with his eyes closed and I sang the songs I had brought. They sat, quietly together and B. died later that day.

It is often the case that however much I plan and consider what an arts session might be, it might, in fact, turn out to be something very different. Again, I have learned that the 'in the moment' flexibility that this requires comes with experience. I have also found that this is something many students need to understand and experience for themselves, as part of their training, so that it does not become a barrier to sustaining paid work once they are qualified. During their placement, students move backwards and forwards between college and hospice. They learn one thing at college and are then often being asked to work in another way at the hospice. Also time constraints and timetables mean that students rarely get the opportunity to attend multi-disciplinary team meetings together with the support and sense of belonging these can bring.

The support that students get from the onsite supervisor is therefore invaluable and can really help mould and prepare competent and realistic practitioners for the future.

I was recently at a multi-disciplinary team meeting at the hospice where we were focussing on a particularly challenging patient. As the meeting went on I listened to the different perspectives that different members of the team brought. There were comments from the social workers, the doctors, the nurses, the health care assistants, the physiotherapist, the psychiatrist and myself as the music therapist. This was a meeting where we explored a range of problems and discovered different opportunities to move forward together. I was really struck by the diversity of the multi-disciplinary team, not just the range of different professionals and perspectives, but also of ages, culture and class, and how this group of people was able to articulate the range of problems that the patient and the family were experiencing, and together began to turn them into opportunities. It was crystal clear that as a multi-disciplinary team, we were able to address the physical, emotional, spiritual and social elements of both the patient's and the family's care.

I am reminded of Colin Murray Parkes, who wrote the following in an annual report of Cruse Bereavement Care:

> We are one people, one community and the death of one is the concern of us all. In the face of death man can achieve grandeur, but if he turns his back on death he remains a child, clinging to a land of make believe. For death is not the ending of the pattern of life's unwinding, but a necessary interruption...there is no easy way through the long valley but we have faith in the ability of each one to find his own way, given time and the encouragement of the rest of us. (p.97)

In this instance, the 'rest of us' is the multi-disciplinary team.

Reflection

Tamsin reminds us that successful team work is an imperative for good quality end of life care, and she supports this fact with some useful examples. Being accepted and becoming an active part of a multi-disciplinary team is not always straightforward, especially when you are not representing in that team what might be thought of as a mainstream health care profession.

I am contacted regularly by artists and arts therapists who work in hospices and other end of life care institutions, and told that they do not feel that they and their work are accepted and valued by either some of the health care professionals they work alongside with or by the organisation they work for as a whole. I think this raises some interesting issues for all of us and it is sometimes too easy not to claim our own responsibility for this.

Respect as a professional is, and should be, hard won. We hear from Tamsin about the challenges and complexities of understanding a range of different professional languages. She also highlights the importance as artists and therapists of honing our language and articulating what we do to the other professionals who we work alongside with in a way that makes sense to them. Her experience of realising that she and the physiotherapist were using the same language – that of structure and rhythm – is an important one. Of course, music moves us physiologically, not just emotionally, and her realisation of this enabled a conversation with the physiotherapist where they could both understand what each other might be offering to the same patient.

One of the strengths of using the arts must surely be that the experience of creating art is not based in everyday language. However, this might lie at the heart of what is most difficult for the arts practitioner when attempting to find a language to talk about what they do. It is also clear that many people do not have the words to talk about such difficult and unusual experiences as death, dying and bereavement. For many, they will also lose the ability to communicate in everyday language due to the progression and nature of their illness. This can lead to feelings of isolation from life and from both established relationships and the possibility of developing new ones. Our relationship, both with ourselves and the world in which we are living and dying, can appear diminished and worthless when we do not have the language or capability to communicate. When life becomes reduced and weakened in this way, it is clear that a variety of opportunities are needed, both to articulate ourselves to ourselves, and also to articulate ourselves to others. Surely, this is where the arts can come into the frame, and without them it is clear that we lack one of the most important tools for people to utilise and engage with when they are feeling isolated and vulnerable.

We know that the creative arts can offer dying people a set of new structures and frameworks in order to understand difficult things, to articulate and confront difficult things and to bring a certain 'order out of chaos'. It is clear from some of the stories that Tamsin shares with us that music and the arts can also give people a new way of collaborating with others. They offer opportunities for patients, family members and carers both to surprise themselves, and to create something which can be left behind as a memory, or more importantly, a legacy. The creative arts provide people with a context where they can be together with others outside of the numbness of illness and outside of incessantly dealing with symptoms of disease and physical problems.

How, as arts practitioners, do we therefore articulate something which does not have its roots in ordinary language to a multi-disciplinary team?

Here, we must remember that talking about what we do is not the same as doing it. Tamsin tells us that it has become clear to her, that one of the only ways of conveying the meaning of her work is to share the music and artwork itself with members of the multi-disciplinary team as part of meetings. This, as well as providing a more concrete example of how the arts work, can also enable the other professionals we work with to see the patient in a new light. As Tamsin says, the team can be surprised and newly motivated by such things as the range of communication skills which might be still available to people, which are witnessed through music and art making, will no longer be evident outside of the structures and frameworks of what the arts can offer.

I can imagine the response of some artists or arts therapists reading this, regarding the importance of respecting patient confidentiality and the professional artists' responsibility of protecting the therapeutic integrity of the music and artworks that are created by patients, family members and carers within arts sessions. This has always puzzled me somewhat. When working as part of a multi-disciplinary team, we are committing ourselves to do the best for our patients and families through working together with the other professionals involved in their care. Most patients and families are aware that their care is down to a team effort and that confidentiality sits within a team framework. We have an obligation to make them aware of this. No one professional should have the responsibility of keeping things to themselves, especially when they can inform other members of the team about something which is important and can affect and influence the work that they too are involved in. If we are keeping things secret regarding our work with patients and families, I would suggest that we need to think seriously about our motivation for doing this. Multi-disciplinary team working is just that. It is about sharing information together with other professionals involved for the benefit of the patients, families and carers we work with. When providing arts or therapy services into hospices or other end of life care organisations, we are part of this sharing network. Our views of working together with patients and families should form part of this sharing, as well as the artwork we have created with them. Sharing the work offers the potential to demystify what the artist or therapist does and gives the potential to share the uniqueness of what this work can bring to people facing death, dying and bereavement with our fellow professionals.

References

Crawford, G.B. and Price, S.D. (2003) 'Team working: palliative care as a model for interdisciplinary practice.' *Medical Journal of Australia 179*, 6, 32.

DH (Department of Health) (2001) *Valuing People.* London: DH.

Hartley, N. and Payne, M. (2008) *The Creative Arts in Palliative Care.* London and Philadelphia, PA: Jessica Kingsley Publishers.

Monroe, B. (2006) 'Team Effectiveness' In P. Speck (ed.) *Teamwork in Palliative Care.* Oxford: Oxford University Press.

Oliviere, D. (2006) 'User Involvement – the Patient and Carer as Team Members?' In P. Speck (ed.) *Teamwork in Palliative Care.* Oxford: Oxford University Press.

Orchard, C.A. and Curran, V. (2003) *Centres of Excellence for Interdisciplinary Collaborative Professional Practice.* Prepared for the Office of Nursing Policy: Health Canada, Government of Canada.

Parkes, C.M. (1984) 'All the End is Harvest.' *The Old Pattern and the New.* London: Darton, Longman & Todd.

Ramsay, N. (2006) 'Sitting Close to Death: a Palliative Care Unit.' In R.D. Hinshelwood and W. Skogstad (eds) *Observing Organisations: Anxiety, Defence and Culture in Health Care.* London: Routledge.

Saunders, C. and Sykes, N. (eds) (1993) *The Management of Terminal Malignant Disease.* 3rd edition. London: Edward Arnold.

Speck, P. (ed.) (2006) *Teamwork in Palliative Care: Fulfilling or Frustrating?* Oxford: Oxford University Press.

Stokes, M. (ed.) (1994) *Ethnicity, Identity and Music.* Oxford and Providence: Berg.

Sutton, J. (2008) *Integrated Team Working: Music Therapy as Transdisciplinary and Collaborative Approaches.* London: Jessica Kingsley Publishers.

Chapter 5

Working with Inpatients

Andy Ridley and Nigel Hartley

Introduction

When St Christopher's Hospice opened in 1967, it was as a large inpatient facility. As has been previously mentioned, there were hospices before St Christopher's, but they were not what we think of as hospices today (Baines 2011). These older hospices, run by a variety of religious orders, provided on-site nursing care for people who were dying, and it is likely that an early focus on inpatient care at St Christopher's was derived from Cicely Saunders' experiences of this much older model (Clark 2002). Although the first ever home care service, which provided dedicated palliative care within the places that people lived, did follow two years later at St Christopher's in 1969, the inpatient unit was initially the main focus of care, with people being admitted and, on the whole, staying until the end of their lives.

With a growth in home care end of life services across the UK over the past 45 years and the increasing emphasis on enabling people to die at home, hospice inpatient units have needed to somewhat change their focus. For example, St Christopher's looks after around 850 people at home on any one day, with an inpatient unit of 48 beds. Although people do still die in hospice inpatient units, it is more than likely that patients will be admitted in crisis, with a focus on resolving the crisis on the inpatient ward, so that they can return home. These crises will range from the complexities of pain and symptom management, to working with family and carer issues, to sorting out serious welfare issues, to supporting someone who is living alone with no informal carers to support them to stay at home. All of this will raise vital challenges when attempting to work therapeutically within an inpatient environment.

Some of these challenges are raised by Andy, who tells us of his experiences of working within an inpatient setting in the hospice. The following headings are addressed:

- The inpatient ward

- St Christopher's Hospice

- Working at the bedside

- Meeting the patient for the first time

- Working with people close to death

- Having started artwork or arts therapy

- Understanding family/carer dynamics, working together with families

- Short-term work, timing and length of sessions

- Working towards discharge into the home or care home, the importance of linking up with community teams.

Andy also includes some case studies to illustrate some key points raised. The chapter ends with my reflection and considerations.

Andy: my background

My name is Andy Ridley and I qualified at Goldsmiths College in 2011 as an arts therapist, with my final student placement being at St Christopher's Hospice. Prior to this I had studied in fine art and photography at university. Although I continued to work on creating my own art, I also worked as a nursing assistant in a large London hospital. Following my placement at St Christopher's I was subsequently offered a job and I presently work there as an art therapist two days a week. It had been difficult qualifying. I failed to pass the course the first time around and spent a year rewriting my final clinical report and re-evaluating my experience as an arts therapist at the hospice. Most of my experience as an art therapy student at St Christopher's was providing one to one art therapy to patients and families on the large inpatient unit. During this time of re-evaluation, I considered training to become a nurse as I had been working for a number of years as a nursing assistant at a large hospital and had continued to do this alongside art therapy training.

What became apparent was that, if I was to qualify and practise as an arts therapist, I needed to acknowledge and reconcile the differences between my training in psychodynamic art, psychotherapy, my concurrent experience as a nursing assistant on an oncology ward and my work as a student arts therapist in a hospice. The tension between therapeutic models and organisational 'best practice' is still with me. It sets the tone and conditions of where I meet patients on a day to day basis at the hospice and how or whether we can work together with art therapy.

The inpatient ward

Working as a nursing assistant on an oncology ward in a large London hospital has helped me understand both the equipment and protocols on the hospice wards, and given me experience in knowing something about the physical needs of patients suffering acute and terminal illnesses.

From my experience, hospital and hospice ward environments are similar. They have similar organisational protocols and hierarchies. On the ward you will find chaplains, complementary therapists, doctors, domestics, nurses, nursing assistants, physiotherapists, psychiatrists, social workers, ward clerks and others, all at various times seeking the attention and co-operation of the patients and those close to them. Multi-disciplinary team meetings are organised to bring staff together to discuss clinical interventions and clinical notes and reports are written on an Electronic Patient Record (EPR) system to report on the details of those interventions and their outcomes. Many of the staff on the ward are doctors or nurses, so it is sometimes easy to feel outnumbered. It has also felt, on occasion, that patients are over-pathologised and that sometimes clinical interventions can be prescriptive in orientation.

On the inpatient ward – for both hospice and hospital – the physical needs of the patient are prioritised. Pain relief, surgical interventions, symptom control, feeding, toileting, personal hygiene and comfort needs are generally administered as soon as is necessary. There are daily nursing routines to accommodate these needs – meal times, medication rounds, washing times – and unlike, for example, arts therapists, the nursing staff are allocated patients on the ward and stay in direct contact with them for the length of each shift. They offer continuity to the patient and are therefore central to the patient's experience of the ward. In short, they become the primary carers of the patient within the hospice and the hospital settings.

Besides the daily routines, the geography of the ward and the equipment and furniture of the ward are also generally there to accommodate the medical and physical needs of the patients. Medication and medical equipment are normally kept on the ward and inpatients eat and drink on the ward and use the toilets if they are able. Patients have bedside chairs and tables, sinks and cupboards and of course, a bed in which to sleep, rest or wait. Many hospice inpatients are bed-bound. At St Christopher's some inpatients have their own room and others stay in bays of four beds. More privacy can be afforded when visiting a patient by pulling closed the curtains around a patient's bed. However, the curtains do not prevent peripheral 'noise' during the arts session or prevent others outside the curtains from hearing what is being said, sung, and so on.

More privacy may certainly be accommodated to those patients in single rooms than those in bays and it may be easier for hospice or hospital staff to maintain patient privacy in a single room. However, there are no emotionally neutral spaces and single rooms might add to feelings of vulnerability and isolation as much as independence and containment for those who stay in them.

Patients are allowed visitors, which means that relatives, friends, staff and others can all be invited to a patient's bedside. Since on both a hospital and hospice ward time is pressing, appropriate times for staff and visitors to be with the patient can become contended. It is within these, often complex, interpersonal and institutional dynamics that arts therapy at a patient's bedside must be negotiated and accommodated.

St Christopher's Hospice

St Christopher's serves a large and culturally diverse population with palliative and end of life care, providing medical and psychosocial support to inpatients on its wards, to day and outpatients in the Anniversary Centre and patients within residential settings. Patients admitted to the wards are generally acutely and terminally ill.

Cicely Saunders was central to establishing modern hospice care. She founded St Christopher's Hospice where she proposed and practised an holistic approach to patient care (Clark 2002). She recognised that dying patients suffer in complex ways and, therefore require 'total' and integrated treatment to ease that suffering. The arts and arts therapies have come to form part of this treatment.

Palliative care is also described as 'patient-led', whereby patients 'have an increased involvement in and responsibility for the circumstances surrounding their own deaths' (Wood 1998b, p.12). Besides medical care, patients might receive arts therapies, creative arts activities, educational, 'reminiscence' and 'life review' work (Hartley and Payne 2008). However, social relationships of power contextualise any therapeutic process (Skaife 1993; Wood 1998a). Patients who come to St Christopher's or any hospice become the subjects of institutional hierarchy, policy and procedure (Evans 2005). The idealised patient is what the staff might make of them – categorised, evaluated and contained (Duesbury 2005; Sontag 1978). Patients can, therefore, easily become passive consumers of assessments, therapies and treatments.

Working at the bedside

Most arts therapists have a designated room or space to which to invite people in for an arts therapy session. This might be a temporary or more permanent space, but it is a space designed to accommodate a creative and therapeutic relationship (Case and Dalley 2006). For inpatients, however, it is often extremely difficult to access and use a designated arts therapy room. With acute and terminally ill bed-bound patients, arts therapists necessarily work at the bedside (Tjasink 2010).

To work on the wards as an arts therapist I use a trolley to carry various art materials to a patient's bedside. Music therapists may take instruments. Occasionally art materials and instruments are left with the patient for personal use or to create work that may be used later with the therapist. At St Christopher's laptops, cameras and recording equipment are also made available for use.

The instruments, art materials and equipment which are taken to the patient help create expectations and limitations on what the patient creates in therapy. It often seems appropriate, with all the interruptions and disruptions on the ward, to try and maintain a sense of continuity to the therapy. However, it is rarely possible, or even appropriate, to see a patient at the same time or on the same day each week. Sometimes I need to see patients daily, and other times we may only meet once. Therefore, having access to the same or similar material for each art or art therapy session may be one way of allowing some continuity and might motivate patients to continue working on the same piece of music or artwork in subsequent sessions.

A hospice ward is emotionally charged. As a visitor one anticipates suffering. We are reminded that our bodies are intimate, sentient and susceptible. For the patient the hospice bed might offer comfort or restraint. It is both a private and public space. Patients are often dressed for bed in pyjamas or nightdresses and connected to catheters, drip-stands and subcutaneous pumps. Protocols regarding infection control must be adhered to. For the artist or arts therapist and particularly for those not medically trained it can be an intimidating place.

Patients may be referred for arts therapy either by the multi-disciplinary team, an individual staff member or a patient's relative or through self-referral. It is good practice to understand the reasons for referral and to ascertain whether the patient is aware of the referral, which is often not the case. The latter can be done prior to meeting the patient by checking the patient records and meeting with the staff member who made the referral. When meeting a patient for the first time it may be appropriate for this staff member to introduce you to the patient. This can help remove the sense of what might be felt as intrusive 'cold calling'.

Clinical assessment and referral for imminently dying patients are necessarily urgent. Patient referrals for arts therapy at St Christopher's are organised formally through an internal EPR system and informally by word of mouth at multi-disciplinary team meetings, at the suggestion of a relative, on ward rounds and elsewhere on site. The group of other artists and arts therapists with whom I work also have formal and informal systems of allocating and 'covering' each referral.

The reasons given for arts or arts therapy referral are as various as the expectations of what it may achieve – 'She seems very bored and listless', 'He used to be a musician', 'He has dysphasia and finds it difficult to express himself', 'It might distract him from the pain', 'I want to make something for my children', 'She read your arts therapy flyer', 'His relative thinks he would benefit from it', 'We want to make something together', 'I want to learn how to draw', to name a few. With such variety, assessments and referrals can often appear random.

This means, when meeting a patient for the first time, the distinction between assessing (or reassessing) patients for arts or arts therapy and offering them arts or arts therapy can be unclear. We – patient and therapist – have to wonder whether something good (or at least not something harmful) may come of the meeting. In my experience, how or whether these expectations are met helps determine the nature of the relationship, at least at the beginning.

To this end, it is important that good relationships are established between artists, arts therapists and the ward nursing staff (Cooper 2006). Understanding and respecting someone's role in the hospice and their relationship to the patient and taking time to explain your own, liaising with staff regarding the patient and reading the patient's notes, enables the artist or therapist to find an appropriate time for the first meeting with the patient and to know something of what to expect. It also allows the artist or therapist to get detailed background information on the patient's social, cultural and medical history, their present condition and emotional state. Different staff members will see arts or arts therapy differently and will refer patients for different reasons. The nurses and nursing assistants in particular form very close relationships with their patients. They are sensitive to the distress patients may be experiencing and might be seeking to comfort them with the arts. The most informed and significant referrals generally come from those who are close to the patient and know something of what the arts or arts therapy can offer them.

Meeting the patient for the first time

Whether introduced to the patient by a staff member or meeting the patient by oneself, it is important for an artist or arts therapist to provide clear information of the service being provided. It might also be necessary to do the same for the patient's family and friends – particularly if they are likely to be present during the session. This information might include questions of confidentiality and safety, the recording of the sessions and the storage and ownership of artworks, the time, duration and frequency of the sessions and the circumstances in which the meetings might be postponed, adapted or ended.

These introductions need to be sensitively handled. How arts and arts therapy is introduced will largely determine how or whether it will proceed and how and when it will end. Often, what is needed from the artist or therapist when introducing the work is both attentiveness to the unique condition of the individual patient and a simple and informal explanation as to what the work offers. Emphasising the range of possible experiences can sometimes make it seem a less foreboding and scary prospect.

Artists and arts therapists know the potential benefits that their work can bring to patients – a more integrated sense of self, a resolve, the realisation of creative expression, a non-verbal or unconscious communication, the learning of a new skill or the re-establishment of an old one, an enhanced recovery, a legacy, a release from anxiety, an emotional respite, and so forth. However, frightened patients with no experience of the arts or therapy will see things differently and may be reluctant to try it. I often find it necessary to persuade the patient of the merits of the arts or arts therapy. I have learned that there is no blueprint here, since each person's experience entering a hospice is different and relationships are uniquely formed and maintained.

Case study: Alison – being gently persistent

Alison had been referred for art therapy informally by a member of her nursing staff. She was an inpatient suffering from terminal cancer. She had respiratory problems and used an oxygen nasal cannula to assist her breathing. She also suffered chest pain, difficulty in swallowing, poor appetite and had severe mobility problems. She was generally confined to her bed or to her bedside chair.

I initially visited her on the ward where she sat, next to her bed in a bay of four beds. Her eyes were closed as if asleep. My intention was to introduce art therapy to her and see whether we thought that might be appropriate for her to try and if so make an appointment to see her later that day.

It felt a little intrusive to call her name but I did. She opened her eyes and despite her politeness, soon seemed impatient for me to leave. I explained quickly and formally who I was and how she might use art therapy but before I could finish she politely and apologetically declined, asking me to come back another day. She said she was tired and in pain. I accepted her explanation without question and left.

The second time I visited Alison she was much the same and she again declined art therapy. And, although she asked me to revisit her another time, it seemed unlikely that art therapy would happen with her.

The third time I saw her was unplanned. As I walked through her ward I noticed that she had been moved to a room of her own. Her door was open and she was sitting next to her bed watching TV. I knocked on the open door and she invited me in. I asked whether she remembered who I was, which she did and I expressed my curiosity at her having moved to a single room. I also noticed a proficiently drawn landscape on her wall, which she explained she had made during a previous hospital stay. Since I did not expect her to want art therapy, my conversation and curiosity was unguarded and informal. Again I invited her to try art therapy and to my surprise, not only did she want to start immediately, she had already decided what she wanted to do. Her first image was to be of Jesus bearing a cross and she wanted to draw his bloodied and broken heart.

From then and over the following four sessions Alison became intensely involved in art therapy. She spoke of the sadness and regret she was re-experiencing at the end of her life and she used her drawing to revisit and re-examine significant moments in her life – both joyous and painful – and to confirm the hope she had invested in her children.

In retrospect, I have no clear idea why Alison was able to engage in art therapy, having twice declined it. Perhaps it was a combination of different things – a temporary improvement in her physical condition; a change in her mental state; the change of environment; a response to my informality on the third visit; or perhaps some contingent factor I am unaware of. Whatever the change, my experience with Alison seemed to show how gently persistent it is necessary to be when offering art therapy to acutely ill patients on the ward.

Leaving flyers with the patient describing the service is perhaps a less imposing introduction to the arts or therapy. Asking those closest to the patient (including the nursing staff) to introduce the work to them may also feel appropriate. However, it is my experience that most inpatients make a decision to start arts or arts therapy after having had a conversation with the artist or arts therapist directly. Patients and therapists need to work one another out. For example, as arts therapists, we are looking to establish a relationship and an environment where it feels safe for the patient to participate. It might be appropriate to offer an introductory session to test the water.

For both artist or therapist and patient, therefore, the first meeting is a crucial indicator of how the relationship may develop. You may be nervous or suspicious or curious of one another. It might feel safe or dangerous, exciting or overwhelming. You will note the physical constraints to working together and whether other people will or should be present during the work that you do together.

It may be important in the first meeting to reflect on this with the patient and where possible talk to others (relatives, nurses, etc.) about your assessment, concerns and intentions with the patient. However, '[i]dentifying those in need of formal therapy can be difficult' (Macleod 2007, p.27). When assessing a patient, we should perhaps remember there are many barriers to engaging in the arts or arts therapy, not least because of the stigma attached to the word 'therapy'. Strand and

Waller (2010) note that older people tend to be more suspicious of something called therapy, associating it with madness.

However, it is also important not to assume everyone needs therapy. Patients often 'have the inherent psychological strengths to manage an incurable illness' (Macleod 2007, p.27). Therefore, arts therapists in particular should try and remain impartial and objective in their assessment of a patient's need and allow patients the autonomy to refuse or accept the service. We are seeking consent and must therefore, be open to the possibility of an immediate start, a deferral or postponement or an outright rejection.

When offering arts or arts therapy to the patient, it is important to be attentive to a patient's initial response to this invitation. Both artists and arts therapists will hear different reasons for declining a referral or informal offer to utilise the arts – 'I am no good at art', 'She is too confused', 'There's no point. I am going to die anyway', 'I am having high-dose chemotherapy', 'Why stir up more trouble?', 'It won't do me any good', 'I am too tired, just now', 'He has enough anxiety as it is', 'That's very kind. Perhaps another time.' When hearing these kinds of responses, we may doubt the reasoning and take it personally – 'I didn't explain it properly', 'The patient is being unnecessarily or neurotically defensive', 'Someone else has decided for the patient.'

It is certainly easier for the artist or therapist to be less doubtful of a patient declining to take part when they hear it directly from them rather than from a third party. But whether from the patient or not, this rejection may be important for the patient to say and the artist or therapist (or any member of staff) to accept. Patients may need gentle persuasion to try out the arts, but I have found from experience that gentle persuasion should remain gentle and not coercive. A useful guide to seeking, making and accepting referrals is perhaps the 'Four Principles' approach presented by Beauchamp and Childress (1994). These are:

1. Respect for autonomy – which recognises the individual's right to decide upon their own destiny and to be in charge of decisions relating to themselves.

2. Benefience – the duty to act in a way that provides benefit to others.

3. Non-malefiance – the duty not to harm.

4. Distributive justice – the fair use and distribution of resources.

Some patients may feel obliged to say yes to the arts or arts therapy, despite themselves. Hospice patients are in a potentially vulnerable and marginalised place. They may feel beholden to or intimidated by family, friends, and sometimes staff. We must, therefore, again be sensitive to the vulnerabilities and dynamics that run through a patient's experience on the ward and make appropriate suggestions on the basis of careful observations and delicate discussions. Having time and experience and confidence in what the arts and arts therapy can offer and bring to people helps.

Whatever the outcome of the first meeting, the medical team are informed of this and clinical notes are concurrently written on the EPR system to keep staff informed of the progress or ending of the artwork and arts therapy.

Working with people close to death

An end of life experience is an intense experience. Despite a biologically 'failing', 'sedated' and 'desensitised' body, all sorts of complex emotional interactions will take place around and with a dying patient. Relief, guilt, hatred, resolve, fatigue, abandonment, love, ambivalence, remorse, disgust, dread, hope might all be felt fleetingly and intensely present, moment by moment. I have found that there is a danger we can be overwhelmed by it all.

The physical manifestation of sickness may also be hard to bear and to witness. A sick body can make us feel sick, reminding us of our own mortality, frailty and susceptibility to illness. A dying body can also sometimes appear contaminated and infectious.

Approaching an acutely ill or dying patient, then, can feel a deeply disturbing prospect. It is a natural response not to want to get too close, emotionally or physically, to a dying person. We might sometimes experience self-preservation before empathy, or over-compensate for our anxieties with inappropriate 'niceness' (Speck 1994).

Having started artwork or arts therapy

Having started artwork or arts therapy on an inpatient unit we must necessarily be open to a range of possible patient engagement both in the art or music making and also in the therapy, dependent on their physical condition. A person's emotional state cannot be separated from their physical condition. Physical impairment and deterioration, fatigue and medication are influential factors in the process and in the relationship that develops. It is therefore important that we are aware of the changing physical conditions of the patient as well as the emotional changes. These physical changes can be observed but also discussed with the patient, the nursing staff and at multi-disciplinary team meetings.

If we are not to deny the arts or arts therapy to end of life patients, we must sometimes assist them in art and music making in ways we would not otherwise do with 'able-bodied' patients. We might be more proactive and directive than we would otherwise be with those who are able-bodied. However, when thinking of such interventions, it is important to take time to reflect upon them. Are we intervening and modifying the conditions appropriately? Or is it that we are we substituting our needs as artists and/or therapists for those of the patient? Is it also possible that such interventions may do more harm than good, for example by disallowing or denying an expression of (or cathartic release from) struggle, frustration, hatred and anger? If we are not to smother, dismiss or passify the dying patient, we must be mindful not to substitute our own 'abilities' for the 'inabilities' of the patient. What might be intended as helpful might be experienced as imposed and alien.

Patient and arts therapist must agree, at least implicitly, on the initial terms and conditions of the work, but also allow for it to be modified at times when appropriate. The therapeutic boundaries, therefore, may hold or shift but will need consideration by the artist and therapist, and need to be reviewed and adapted when necessary with the patient's consent.

What happens at the end of the work will also need some thought. When working with a dying patient, it is understandably tempting for the patient and artist to avoid discussions around the ending or interrupting the work – both the ending of each session and the ending of work as a whole. However, endings and interruptions are unavoidable in this environment. With dying patients in a hospice, work is often interrupted and endings are unpredictable. A patient may suffer acute pain during the time you are with them and need medication to alleviate it. Patients often become very tired and fall asleep or ask to stop the work in order to sleep. The patient may be discharged before the art sessions have been completed. Also, of course, the patient may physically deteriorate to the point where they are no longer able to engage in the work being done.

It often seems both patient and artist or therapist have little control over the ending of the work. And because an intensely felt relationship is often formed, its loss through the death of the patient can be difficult to manage. Leaving the patient after each session can feel like abandonment. Stopping the work all together due to a patient's physical deterioration or change of circumstance can be scarring. Processing the ending to the work you do together therefore requires good supervision and support.

Whether or not the patient is discharged or dies, decisions will have to be made as to the artworks and recordings which have been created. Are they to be stored at the hospice, destroyed or given to a patient or next of kin? Has this been discussed with the patient or relatives? Is confidentiality being breached if artworks are offered to a third party?

The legacy of the artwork and the fate of the things produced within it need to be considered in the light of the patient and their relative's wishes prior to their discharge or death and the legal frameworks governing such decisions. When a patient dies, grieving relatives may naturally need time to make decisions regarding a patient's artworks or musical recordings made during the work you have done with them. Delaying a decision is often appropriate at this stage.

Understanding family/carer dynamics, working together with families

When people become hospice inpatients their relationships with others change. Relatives, friends and loved-ones come to the ward to offer comfort and company but in the context of an unfamiliar environment. Visitors may have shared a long personal history with the patient prior to admission. They may have been the primary caregiver. When a patient is admitted onto the ward, those close to them must necessarily abrogate at least some responsibility for the wellbeing of the patient (onto the staff at the hospice). For some this may be difficult and for others this may be a burden lifted.

Whatever the changes in the relationship, those close to the patient may want to remain close to them on the ward. This might also be what the patient wants. A connectedness can be maintained either face to face or using mobile phone or computer-aided technology (such as Skype), but with increasing frailty and physical impairment, patients and those close to them are reminded of the finiteness of their relationships and may want to spend as much time together as possible.

Ward staff, therefore, must often be aware of and sensitive to these relationships and how they are maintained and adapted. It is my experience that patients and family members sometimes insist on a family member or members staying with the patient during an arts or arts therapy session – particularly the first one. Sometimes this 'third party' may actively participate in the work and even be central to it, for example, by singing or playing an instrument or making artwork alongside the patient or by being involved in a three or more-way conversation.

The presence and participation of a 'third party' can also lead to a potentially complex and dynamic, emotional experience. In this situation, the art can often feel unfocussed. With other people around, the patient might also seem to be marginalised and otherwise self-censoring. We can experience jealousies and divided loyalties from and towards the patient.

However, it is also my experience that creating art with others present beside the patient, rather than being limited, can lead to quite profound moments of validation and self-realisation for all those involved. What we can often experience in this situation is a relationship in the making or perhaps the confirmation or validation of an earlier one.

Case study: Maria's portrait of her daughter

I initially met Maria when she had participated in an art group while an inpatient at St Christopher's. She was an English-speaking, Italian woman in her 60s who had brought generosity and humour to the group and had taken to portraiture with growing enthusiasm. We had also had had a one to one art therapy session on the ward when she had once been too weak to join the group. She had widespread, metastatic cancer and her prognosis was poor. After a few weeks in the hospice she became visibly weaker and drawn and as her health and mobility deteriorated, we agreed to meet for another one to one art therapy session on the ward.

By the time we met, Maria's adult daughter was spending every day with Maria and she asked to stay with her mother during art therapy. Maria welcomed the idea and in fact, decided she would draw a portrait of her daughter in the session. She chose to use pencils and drew slowly and deliberately but with great affection and playfulness. There were many moments of tenderness between them both.

Halfway through the drawing and the session Maria paused and said that she was lost. She did not elaborate and after some quiet reflection continued with the drawing and her engagement with her daughter.

By the end of the session Maria felt her drawing to be complete and both Maria and her daughter enjoyed the accomplishment. I asked to take the drawing with me, temporarily, to look at and think about and arranged our next meeting.

Later that same day Maria's daughter stopped me on the ward and gently probed me for information regarding her mother's medical prognosis. Maria was to be discharged within the next few days to her family home. I described what physical changes I had noticed but talked mainly of what I had noticed of them both during the earlier art session. I suggested she consult her medical team for information regarding Maria's physical health and wellbeing.

I returned to Maria a few days later, on the day she was due to be discharged. I wanted to say goodbye and discuss Maria's drawing, what it meant to her and what she wanted to do with it. We agreed that to protect it from damage, I would photograph it and then send it to her via email. She was proud to have made it and for it to have been recognised as something beautiful. She looked forward to going home and being with her family again. The drawing would be something she could share with them.

Maria died two weeks after discharge. I waited a few weeks after her death before contacting Maria's daughter. She had received her mother's drawing and she thanked me for it and for the pleasure she remembered feeling with her mother as she had made it.

Although our focus is normally on the patient and their needs, it is often also important at the same time to be sensitive to the needs of others close to the patient such as their family members or friends. This requires open, honest and sensitive communication among all those concerned. These people may need reassurance and information regarding the arts services and the artist or arts therapist may need to discuss and decide with them the most appropriate times for the work to happen. If this is done with consideration and care and with the knowledge and co-operation of the patient, it is likely there will be less disruption to the art sessions and less conflict surrounding them before, during and after therapy has ended. It may also mean there is less suspicion of the therapist and of the 'therapy' in 'arts therapy'.

For the arts work to continue, an artist or arts therapist must allow for, and work with, the various and changing physical conditions of the patient and their altering peripheral circumstances while also attempting to maintain a place in which to work creatively together. In order not to feel overwhelmed by these changing conditions and to begin to make sense of the artwork being done and the changes within the relationship, it is essential that artists and arts therapists are able to reflect upon and process the work through peer review, multi-disciplinary team meetings and clinical supervision. We also need to know our limitations and work with them. There are no perfect conditions to using the arts anywhere in health and social care, and this is particularly so in end of life care. Time is short and the environment is often busy, cluttered and messy. As artists and therapists, we try and get what we can, when we can. We work with unconscious and complex emotional interactions. With experience, we make time to think about and process the work we do and find other experienced people to help us to do that as well as possible.

Short-term work, timing and length of sessions

Almost without exception, arts work on a hospice ward is brief. Patients can die or be discharged with no or little warning after a short stay on the ward. Single sessions are not unusual and the ending to the work is often abrupt and unpredictable.

In this context it can be tempting to compensate for the brevity and imminent ending by trying to 'speed things up'. It becomes tempting for the artist to offer immediate interpretation and meaning to the patient's experiences. Surely we should offer, like the medical team, immediate and unconditional solace and comfort to those who are so obviously suffering? To wait for the patient to find meaning in their end of life experience can feel unbearable, especially when this meaning might be buried deep in an unconscious, physically impaired and non-verbal experience. How are we both, patient and artist/ therapist, to tolerate such potential loss and uncertainty?

It often feels as an art therapist that I do not know what I am supposed to do with a dying patient. It can feel voyeuristic and perverse to be with them. Am I to facilitate a search for meaning? To act as witness? To validate creative expression? To tolerate and contain psychic pain or hateful projection? To allow for cathartic release? To improve cognitive faculty and co-ordination? To create a legacy? To help normalise death? Or is indeed my being with them more to do with some externally imposed criteria, like me validating my own role on the ward?

Having such questions and insecurities and questioning the purpose of the creative arts and arts therapies might be a reflection of similarly felt insecurities the patient may be experiencing, and the insecure and changing institutional, cultural and social frameworks concerning death and dying that inform the patient's experience. They may also reflect unresolved ideas of what it means to be a 'good' member of staff in a 'caring profession'. Our questions and insecurities derive from the sometime conflicting, clinical, ethical, legal, experiential and unconscious considerations.

With so much potential insecurity, perhaps the most difficult task for an arts therapist (or for any member of staff at a hospice) is knowing when and how to allow for ambivalence and ambiguity in a therapeutic relationship – to sit with the flow and exchange of things – a love and/or hate, a sureness and/or doubt, a hope and/or horror.

As an arts therapist I am trained to work with deeply felt, unconscious emotions. Different training and schools of thought inform the approach and attitude towards the patient and the art therapy. Sometimes the experience of art therapy seems to fit a therapeutic model. Most times, however, it does not.

There is much we do not know and will never know of the dying experience and this not-knowing often feels unbearable. If, as artists and therapists, we choose to work with patients in palliative and end of life care, we must find ways of living and working with those doubts. Our own experience and the experience of others shows that there is always a chance we might respond appropriately and ease their pain.

Working towards discharge into the home or care home, the importance of linking up with community teams

It might be generally assumed that most patients admitted as inpatients to a hospice will die there, but in reality many inpatients are discharged. If the patient is discharged while in the middle of some artwork or arts therapy, it is often the case that the work can continue within the patient's home or other residential setting.

If this happens, arrangements must be made with the patient and others responsible for the patient's care. What may have been appropriate and possible as an inpatient may not necessarily be appropriate or possible in another setting. The patient may live too far from the hospice either to visit the hospice as an outpatient or be visited by the artist or arts therapist. There may be other extenuating circumstances that make it impossible to continue working together. It might also be that the artwork and/or therapy, in parallel with the treatment plan at the hospice, has simply run its course.

However the work ends and whenever possible, thought should be given as to what to do with the artworks and recordings which have been made by the patient. Some patients may want all or some of the work made to be given to family members or friends. Other patients may want to keep all or some of their work (or reproductions of it) for themselves, while others will not care either way.

Artworks can embody powerful feelings and memories. They last over time and can represent a continuity of feeling when much else for a sick person might seem fractured and unpredictable. If patients return to the arts or arts therapy after a break, previous artwork and recordings can offer a bridge to new work being created.

It is also possible that the work continues in a different setting after discharge. If not in the hospice as an outpatient, this will be in a residential setting. This development will need careful planning and co-operation primarily with the patient, but also with respect to all those involved in the patient's continued care.

A new setting may require new approaches and new ways of thinking about the work you do together. Presupposed parameters may need reconsideration. Questions of confidentiality and the timing and length of the meetings in this new environment will need some thought, and the new environment may limit what art materials and instruments are used. If the patient is discharged to a care home, the artist or therapist will need to talk to the management of the care home to ensure there is no harmful conflict of interest regarding the work taking place.

In these new circumstances it is often the case that feeding back to the multi-disciplinary team at the hospice takes on a greater significance, since the artist may be, for the patient, one of the only direct or regular points of contact with the hospice after the patient is discharged.

I have focussed on the institutional dynamics and the material context that frame arts work and arts therapy work on a hospice ward. It is meant as a practical guide but it can never be definitive. Hospices and their protocols may vary, and different artists and arts therapists will bring different approaches and models, different expectations, expertise and experience to the patients they work with.

Assessing and reassessing one's work and the environment in which it is practised is often difficult and therefore requires thorough and consistent supervision and peer support, even for the most experienced of artists and arts therapists.

Also, if we are to practise safely and consistently as artists or arts therapists, it is not only important to be aware of the external conditions to the work, but also to maintain and extend our self-awareness. Artists and therapists will be affected by their dying patients. We are with them through difficult times and can often feel overwhelmed and inadequate. For our continued wellbeing and so as not to reflect and reinforce the anxieties of the patient, we must recognise and process the grief and insecurity we experience as people who work in end of life care through continually developing the awareness we have of both ourselves and the work that we do (through, for example, supervision, personal therapy, etc.). By doing this, we might help set the preconditions where the arts and arts therapy can be a fruitful experience for all those involved.

Reflection

Working on an inpatient ward at the bedside of someone who is extremely physically ill poses a set of very specific challenges. These challenges range from understanding the complexities of the health environment in which we are working, navigating our way through a set of professional relationships with doctors and nurses, as well as understanding the intricacies of family dynamics and how we articulate what we do to everyone involved, which will include the patient with whom we are intending to work. In many ways, Andy comes to work as an arts therapist on an inpatient ward with a unique set of experiences. He tells us that he has already worked as a nursing assistant on an acute oncology hospital ward for many years. This experience furnishes him with a knowledge of and familiarity with how inpatient care works. He knows the environment, the equipment he can expect to come across, the different types of health care professionals he will encounter and something of what both patients and their families will be living through. However, he has not yet worked as an artist in this setting, and he explains to us some of the particular issues that this raises for him. He quickly realises that working as a nursing assistant and an arts therapist are two very different things, even though the environment he encounters is familiar. He has to rethink and re-establish a set of working relationships which are going to be useful to him as part of a new and different role.

Although Andy comes to the hospice with his specific set of experiences, for many artists, this will not be the case. In this situation, the danger will be that the inpatient ward will become forbidden territory and that using the arts within this kind of setting will be seen as either irrelevant or inappropriate. In my own experience, I have often had the feeling that the inpatient unit can be seen to be 'hallowed ground', the place where the 'real work' happens. It will be important to work through this issue and beyond it as quickly as possible, particularly if the arts are to be seen as relevant and useful as part of the care of patients within such an environment. It might be worth arranging to work a couple of shifts as a volunteer or nursing assistant on the inpatient ward, familiarising yourself with the context as well as focussing on establishing the relationships with key staff which Andy mentions.

I always think that patients and their families receiving care and support from an inpatient ward will be expecting to see a doctor or a nurse, and these roles will be immediately recognisable to them, either through the identification of uniforms or the medical equipment which is utilised. We must realise that approaching a patient and/ or their family as a musician or artist, however, will be an alien experience for most people. Approaching a patient who is in their bed for the first time with a guitar or a set of paints, for example, might be completely bewildering to them, even terrifying. It is not surprising, therefore, that an artist or arts therapist might be sent away by the patient or family member with a 'flea in their ear'. Andy talks of the sensitivity and humility needed when working within an inpatient environment, and this involves careful consideration of how the arts and arts therapies can be presented and articulated; not only to members of the multi-disciplinary team, but also to the patients and family members themselves.

I have had many experiences of working with patients at their bedsides on an inpatient ward. I would describe some of these experiences as having been complex, intense and even life-changing. However, I have sometimes been caught short when being too self-laudatory. Once, I had spent a long period time with a gentleman writing and recording a song to be played at his funeral. The experience had been challenging and powerful and had stayed with me for a number of days. When I returned with a copy of the recording to give to him, he grabbed hold of my arm and said 'Thank God you have come!' He then went on to ask for two chocolate bars from the sweets trolley as he wanted to give them to his grandchildren who were visiting later that day. In reality, he had somehow thought that I was one the volunteers who regularly came around selling drinks and sweets. I found the trolley and sold him two chocolate bars and nothing more was said. I asked one of the nurses to pass on the recording to him, which was played at his funeral two weeks later. Relationships within an intense, highly-charged environment can sometimes be full of twists and turns. In reality, my experience shows that people need us to be the person they need us to be at different times; at one time someone who can support them to write their song to be played at their funeral, and at another time someone who can sell them chocolates to give to their grandchildren. Both should be possible. If we cannot be who they want us to be, with a minimum of fuss, we should easily be able to call on another member of the team to support them and help them out.

To conclude, Andy also raises another most important issue, that of the tension that sometimes exists between the training institutions and the student's placement organisations. There can sometimes be a gap that exists between what we train art or art therapy students to do and what, in reality, is needed within a series of potential workplaces (Hartley 2008). For example, teaching a music therapy student that individual sessions should take place on a weekly basis for the same amount of time, normally 50 minutes, within a designated room, is all very well in theory. However, when working in a hospice or similar end of life care institution, this will never or rarely be the case. A student can be left feeling bewildered and also believing themselves to be a failure when they discover that the reality of day to day work as an artist or arts therapist is entirely different from what they have been led to believe back at college. This can also be the case for newly qualified artists or arts therapists when stepping into working in a variety of health care settings for the first time. I have seen a number of new artist and arts therapies posts fall at the first hurdle due to expectations and realities not being matched. A sense of mistrust might therefore be established which can never be mended.

There is still much work to be done in realigning what we teach artists and therapists to do in health care, and what is needed in actuality. After all, the landscape of health care changes continuously, and we should be teaching and preparing our future health care practitioners to deliver services in ways that organisations and their users want and need as part of a changing landscape as opposed to explaining to them a set of theoretical models which may have been established as part of a different age and now may not always be useful or even relevant.

References

Baines, M. (2011) St Christopher's Hospice website. www.stchristophers.org.uk, accessed on 12 June 2013.

Beauchamp, T.L. and Childress, J.F. (1994) *Principles of Biomedical Ethics*. New York: Oxford University Press.

Case, C. and Dalley, T. (2006) *The Handbook of Art Therapy*. Hove: Routledge.

Clark, D. (2002) *Cicely Saunders, Founder of the Hospice Movement. Selected Letters 1959–1999*. Oxford: Oxford University Press.

Cooper, J. (ed.) (2006) *Stepping into Palliative Care 1: Relationships and Responses*. 2nd edition. Oxford: Radcliffe Publishing.

Duesbury, T. (2005) 'Art Therapy in the Hospice: Rewards and Frustrations.' In D. Waller and C. Sibbett (eds) *Art Therapy and Cancer Care*. New York: Open University Press.

Evans, K. (2005) 'On Death and Dying.' In D. Waller and C. Sibbett (eds) *Art Therapy and Cancer Care*. New York: Open University Press.

Hartley, N. (2008) 'The arts in health and social care – is music therapy fit for purpose?' *British Journal of Music Therapy 22*, 2, 88–96.

Hartley, N. and Payne, M. (2008) *The Creative Arts in Palliative Care*. London and Philadelphia, PA: Jessica Kingsley Publishers.

Macleod, S. (2007) *The Psychiatry of Palliative Medicine: The Dying Mind*. Oxford and New York: Radcliffe Medical Press.

Skaife, S. (1993) 'Sickness, health and the therapeutic relationship: Thoughts arising from the literature on art therapy and physical illness.' *International Journey of Art Therapy: Inscape*. Summer, 24–29.

Sontag, S. (2003) *Regarding the Pain of Others*. London: Penguin Books.

Speck, P. (1994) 'Working with Dying People.' In A. Obholzer *et al.* (eds) *The Unconscious at Work: Individual and Organisational Stress in the Human Services*. London: Routledge.

Strand, S. and Waller, D. (2010) 'The experience of Parkinson's: Words and images through art therapy – a pilot research study.' *International Journey of Art Therapy: Inscape 15*, 2, 84–93.

Tjasink, M. (2010) 'Art psychotherapy in medical oncology: a search of meaning.' *International Journey of Art Therapy: Inscape 15*, 2 December.

Wood, M.J.M. (1998a) 'Art Therapy in Palliative Care.' In M. Pratt and M.J.M. Wood (eds) (1998) *Art Therapy in Palliative Care*. London and New York: Routledge.

Wood, M.J.M. (1998b) 'What is Palliative Care?' In M. Pratt and M.J.M. Wood (eds) (1998) *Art Therapy in Palliative Care*. London and New York: Routledge.

Chapter 6

Working with Day and Outpatients

Mick Sands and Nigel Hartley

Introduction

The central part of this chapter introduces us to Mick. Mick is a community artist working in end of life care. He tells us something about himself, and of his personal experience of working with day patients, outpatients and their families and carers. The following areas are addressed:

- Hospice day care: some background

- Day care models

- What kind of professional groups do we encounter in day care?

- Volunteers

- Working as a community artist in day care: some personal thoughts

- Working with individuals

- Working with groups

- Exhibitions and performances.

The background to end of life day care is explored and various models are introduced and explained. The strengths and weaknesses of current end of life day care models are highlighted and examined, and relevant recent research and evaluation studies which have scrutinised service delivery and offered guidance for future development are included.

As a context which lends itself to group work possibilities, Mick gives an example of planning and running a group within the day care context. This is focussed around the St Christopher's Schools Project, which is a dynamic health promotion project bringing in local school children and students to work alongside dying people and their families. Some key considerations are also given when working one to one with users. Although it is likely that volunteers will be encountered in many end of life care contexts, particularly within hospices, a section gives various perspectives on the roles of the volunteer within this particular environment and offers guidance on how volunteers can be utilised as a help as part of your own work.

Mick adds two stories to support his experiences and the chapter ends with my reflection. As part of this reflection, I also share the story of the development and execution of a new day care and outpatient facility at St Christopher's Hospice, London known as the Anniversary Centre. This acts as an example of a response to some of the changes and challenges that Mick raises for this particular end of life care context.

Mick: my background

My name is Mick Sands and I work as a freelance musician and theatre composer. Just over five years ago I took up a part-time post as a community artist at St Christopher's Hospice. I had an instinct that this was an appropriate creative pathway for me and would give me an opportunity to combine my past experiences in order do something quite new and unique.

I come from a family of singers and a tradition of people singing together. I was involved in the Folksong Revival in the 1960s and performed with my brothers and sister as a way of exploring my Irish cultural roots. At boarding school I had choral training and learned about instrumental music. I went on to do an English degree, trained and began work as a secondary education teacher while continuing to sing and perform with amateur theatre groups and street theatre companies.

As time went on, I became very involved with a charity for adults with learning disabilities. I left the teaching profession and began to train in counselling and dramatherapy. At this time, I began to weave my music and drama interests into work with disabled adults and children. One of the things I enjoyed most was co-founding and managing a craft workshop with disabled adults within a residential community in South London. My own personal therapy has also been an important part of my personal development, particularly analytical psychotherapy of which the use of art was a significant part. I had always drawn and painted and had an interest in art and art history. When I left the charity I taught part time, working with statemented pupils in secondary education. I also worked as a musician and coached actors in singing. My voice work took me into the professional theatre and I began adapting and then finally composing music for classical plays. I have worked in many of the major theatre companies across the UK over the past 25 years. Such work, however, has been irregular and I continue to work as composer/musician/performer in a variety of settings. The part-time community artist post at St Christopher's has provided some stability within the sporadic nature of the rest of my work.

My personal and professional life has been wide-ranging and eclectic but almost exclusively concerned with the expressive, creative arts. Those I have worked alongside have included students, fellow artists and people for whom I have had a duty of care.

My journey to this work has been directed by a need to make a living and a desire to do what I enjoy. I continuously experience a certain ambivalence about whether to pursue my own work to make a living, to continue finding my own creative voice or to develop my skills as an artist in the service of others. My experience tells me that there is no simple answer, and my work is a mix of many different motivational properties. On good days I have a sense of joy and fulfilment in all of my many work strands, and during these times it all seems marvellous good fortune. On not-so-good days I feel inadequate, lacking orthodoxy and a clear label to describe myself. On these days, I can even feel that I am some kind of imposter.

Hospice day care: some background

Most hospices in the UK will have a day care programme, as will many other end of life care organisations such as some hospitals and care homes. In fact, in hospices alone, there are around 220 day centres across the country. Hospices added day care centres as a service that their users benefit from when they began to develop themselves more widely during the mid-1970s. On the whole, these day centres based themselves on a pre-existing model of geriatric day care services

(Fisher and McDaid 1996). This is mainly defined by being available between 10am and 3pm during some or all weekdays. From an older person's perspective, one can see and understand that allowing time in the morning to get up and prepare for the day, as well as leaving time later in the day for any necessary care to be given at home before going to bed, is a sensible idea. From a content point of view, most day care centres for older people provide meals, social opportunities and recreational outings, as well as more general supervision. In some centres, a nurse is employed to provide necessary checks on people's conditions, and some research studies highlight that one of the benefits of day care is the prevention of hospitalisation, enabling the person to live to the best of their capacity within their own home (Copp *et al.* 1998). Another major area of benefit highlighted within research studies of day care provision for older people is for carers. While their family member is attending day care, they are given much needed time to themselves to either recuperate from their intensive caring role or to undertake necessary jobs which are not possible during their normal caring regime. Preventing hospitalisation and providing respite to carers were also key to the early developmental aims of many end of life care day centres (Hearn and Myers 2001). It is also important to know that many day care centres in hospices were also initiated by existing professionals. What is meant by this is that maybe a nurse who had worked on the inpatient ward, or an occupational therapist who had worked between the inpatient ward and the community, developed an interest in establishing a day care service in order to address some of the issues that they had encountered during their work. They then took up the remit of researching into and setting up a day care service. It is clear that the model of day care that was created was based around the professional competences of the person setting it up (Fisher and McDaid 1996). If that person was a nurse, it is likely that the service would be based in the first instance around addressing the nursing needs of the people who used the service, with other elements such as social or group work possibilities being added at a secondary level. Similarly if the person setting up the service came from an occupational therapy background, group work and occupational activities would be given centre stage, while nursing might be absent, or at best seen as a supporting role.

Day care models

There has been a criticism that many day care services were not necessarily founded and developed based on patient need, but on the interests, enthusiasms and agendas of those who set them up and then ran them (Fisher and McDaid 1996). This kind of instigation led to the embodiment of a number of what have become known as hospice day care 'models'. This list normally includes the following:

- *Medical model* – this includes the possibility for medical interventions such as blood transfusions or other treatments to be available and administered on a daily basis.

- *Nursing model* – an example of this would be when the patients who attend day care have their nursing needs met in that context as opposed to being visited at home by a community nurse specialist.

- *Psychosocial or social model* – this type of day centre would offer a programme to meet the psychological or social needs of those attending. This might include a variety of one to one therapies or group possibilities.

It could be argued that end of life day care centres, which were set up as part of hospices based on Cicely Saunders' concept of 'total pain' and aspiring to treat 'the whole person' (Clark 2002) might fail to live up to that promise. For example, a patient attending a social model of day care, who was feeling unwell and could benefit from some nursing input, might be excluded for this reason, needing to stay at home for a nurse to visit them there.

As well as being defined by a specific and limited time frame with availability being between 10am and 3pm during the week, day care centres are also limited by 'context'. The centres will generally revolve around one large room where those who attend spend most of their time together. The large room will only be able to hold a certain number of people, and the size of the room will limit the number of people who can attend and therefore be referred to the service. On the whole, end of life day care centres in the UK offer places for between 10 and 30 people a day. On average about two thirds of those booked actually attend due to the fact that many people might not feel well enough, or have other priorities such as hospital appointments or home visits by community health and social care professionals

(Hearn and Myers 2001). This style of day care is also only attractive to a percentage of people. For example, on average about one quarter of any hospice patient population take up attendance at the day care service (Douglas *et al.* 2003). If a hospice or end of life care unit looks after a patient population of 400 across the community it serves, it is therefore likely that around 100 of those patients will accept a referral to day care. This is for a number of reasons. First, it is very difficult to 'sell' day care to some patients. Most of them will have a fantasy or an image of a group of people sitting around in a circle playing games or being entertained. Second, it is common that many patients will be afraid to attend the hospice building. It is clear that if day care is not your scene, there are very few other possibilities to offer social or therapeutic experiences or interaction with others. Indeed, many day care centres, by the very nature of the model and style that they embrace, do exclude certain types of people (Douglas *et al.* 2003).

What kind of professional groups do we encounter in day care?

Professional groups utilised by day care centres will include:

- nurses: community nurse specialists, registered nurses and heath care assistants

- a variety of therapists who will include a range of allied health professionals such as physiotherapy, occupational therapy and arts therapies

- artists and arts therapists (paid staff and/or volunteers)

- chaplain or spiritual care lead

- social workers

- complementary therapists (paid staff and/or volunteers)

- volunteers – offering general support.

As already mentioned, some centres will have nursing teams who will offer hands-on nursing care when needed in order to reduce the need for home visits by community nurse specialists. Other centres will employ a 'token' nurse, who will be there to offer security should anyone become unwell during the day. These particular nurses might have opted out of mainstream nursing in order to develop and practise their interest in social or therapeutic work. Health care assistants may also be employed in some day care centres in order to offer more basic nursing care such as changing dressings or bathing patients.

Most day centres will have access to a medical team in some way. It is common either for doctors to be available in an emergency, or for a named, usually junior, doctor to carry the responsibility for day care patients.

Volunteers

Volunteers have been an important part of the delivery of end of life care since the outset. Cicely Saunders wrote that St Christopher's Hospice enrolled the first volunteer before the first patient was admitted (Clark 2002). Hospices in particular have utilised volunteers in a number of ways. It is common to come across volunteers helping and supporting with fundraising events, and also giving their time to help run the hundreds of hospice charity shops across the country. In terms of volunteers working directly with patients and carers, there are opportunities for volunteers to support users on inpatient wards, in day care centres and also in the home. Most bereavement services also make use of specially trained volunteers to support people through the bereavement process. In terms of user-facing volunteers, many organisations will run training programmes in order to equip them with the skills and knowledge needed in order to be of help to those coming to the end of life.

However, it is important to be aware that some organisations do not offer any formal training for volunteers. When they do, volunteers' training programmes vary greatly from organisation to organisation, with some offering a fairly intense training course before the volunteer can begin and others offering a few key sessions after volunteers have started. On the whole, volunteers will provide hospitality and basic, practical support to users within the major contexts mentioned. In general, volunteers in the UK contribute around £46 billion to the economy, with over a 100,000 volunteers supporting hospices alone (Doyle 2002). Some of the key benefits include the fact that they bring to organisations a variety of community representation and help and also the message they take back out into the community to normalise death and dying and to help to change public perceptions of the work that hospices do.

On another note, many people will volunteer their time to a hospice because of having a personal experience of a friend or family member having died under the care of the organisation. Although this motivation is understandable, on occasions it can provide a number of challenges. One of these might be around the different expectations a volunteer and the organisation might have. During the process of witnessing the quality of care received by both a friend or relative, it might be surprising that this experience changes when they become a volunteer. This will not be because volunteers are treated badly by organisations, but because the experience of being a volunteer within an organisation will differ greatly from that of being a user of services. Many volunteers may not be prepared for this change of focus, however subtle the change might be. There can also be problems with some volunteers and the length of time they might continue to volunteer with an organisation. We all know that it is difficult to accept change when we have become used to things being done in certain ways over long periods of time. It is not unusual for hospices to report the difficulties they are experiencing with volunteers who do not understand change and actively resist it.

This tension is very evident during current times, as many hospices find new ways of responding to current social and economic pressures. It is likely that the volunteer contribution within end of life care will grow and become more important, as organisations reform their volunteer procedures and processes in order to meet the current gaps and deficits that we witness in both health and social care.

It is common to come across volunteers in day centres who will provide what some might call 'professional services'. For example, people who are qualified as complementary therapists, have an interest in the creative arts, hairdressers, beauticians and religious leaders all volunteer their time within many end of life day care centres. It will be common, and can be very useful, that a volunteer might support paid artists when running groups within day care centres. Also, in some centres, volunteers will run arts groups by themselves. When this is the case, it is important to be clear regarding qualifications to practise and professional registration. It is also important to realise that just because someone might be qualified to practise a certain role, this does not mean that they will necessarily be suitable to offer their skills within end of life care. Training will be equally important for these people, in order to establish parity with both other volunteers and paid members of staff.

Working as a community artist in day care: some personal thoughts

My daily personal and professional challenge is to be compassionate and respectful. The way we come into relationships with those who are dying and their families, carers and communities is most important to me. I have learned the importance of validating and respecting both them and their experiences and accepting that they are, in fact, the experts on themselves. I know that we need to be mindful of their health as well as their illness and to relate to them as whole people with many facets and strands to the narratives of their lives. I always seek to make an alliance with them through using the arts, creating open and healthy possibilities between us. I believe in maintaining an awareness of our transactions with care and with honesty, taking note of all the communications, verbal and non-verbal, the sounds and marks made, noticing the metaphorical, the conscious and unconscious communications. Such observations are all part of the tool set to help increase our understanding of the person and their situation, and with this we take our place in a multi-disciplinary palliative care service, helping the patient to 'live until they die'.

I believe that the act of making music, of forming clay, of putting paint on canvas, of writing poetry, of singing or playing a musical instrument can express the range and detail of our physical, emotional, spiritual and intellectual lives. My experience has shown me that the process of doing these art activities can be both highly enjoyable and painfully difficult, and can lead to a fuller sense of ourselves. I have also learned that the outcomes of these activities can be valued aesthetically and valued because of what they release in the person who made them. To interpret Cicely Saunders' words 'You matter because you are you' (Clark 2002), therefore your art matters because it is your art. My work as a community artist entails working with outpatients, with patients in daycare, one to one sessions, group work, health promotion, setting up exhibitions, performances, being in an arts team and working with other professionals. The people I come into contact with are living with a terminal illness. They might be having curative medical treatment or undergoing procedures to slow its progression and manage its symptoms. They might have issues with pain, or increasing disability through the spread of the disease. The burden of managing the disease on themselves, their carers and family might be significant. Their social skills might be affected, leading to loneliness and isolation in their community. Their mood might be low because of such pressures: worrying about the future, how they and their families will cope financially and emotionally. They might be afraid and low in confidence. They might be angry and bitter that such a thing has happened to them. They might still be in shock of first diagnosis, in denial that their illness is terminal or grieving the loss of life as they knew it. They might be doing well but would simply appreciate meeting other people 'in the same boat'.

Working with individuals

The terminal nature of a patient's illness means they are going through an inevitable process of change, often unpredictable, sometimes rapid, sometimes tedious and slow, marked by fluctuating 'wellness' and 'illness', and this is normal and natural. There may be limited opportunities to work, sometimes there's a sense of not having much time, of time being short. I have learned that we have to be opportunists and at the same time carry our expectations lightly; be aware that we are dealing with endings, with closure, at the same time looking for ways to acknowledge and affirm their creative vitality.

I realise as I write this how difficult I find the concept of 'short-term' work. My personality type wants to keep exploring the options and play with possibilities. It also connects to my own fear of death. For example, I sometimes find it difficult to bring a series of sessions to a close. That can be compounded when the patient also does not want them to end. Endings can be difficult but they are a normal part of life. They can also make other things possible. Sudden, unexpected endings do occur. Death or sudden disease deterioration can mean that it is no longer possible to meet with the patient. One is left with a whole mix of emotions. The relief of knowing that their fears, anxiety, whatever they were suffering, are over. Guilt at missing an opportunity to respond and of not having done enough. Sometimes I am angry, disappointed, and feel cheated that something was not completed; my sense of satisfaction has been interrupted, and the intensity and intimacy created in the work have gone. Sometimes I have an acute sense of loss. It is a process of grieving that I accept is a vital part of our work.

It is important to be focussed and clear about the purpose of the work that we are engaged in. It can sometimes be helpful to agree a concrete outcome, a target, something that we can discuss, evaluate together, and celebrate; there is something about coming to the end of creating products together that is an important part of our practice. It might be 'to make something as a legacy for my children or grandchildren' or 'to make something that might help me to cope with the difficult days that lie ahead'. It might be simply: 'let's spend some time playing with clay' or 'let's sing some of your favourite songs'.

Another purpose of engaging with the dying person and their family is to discover strategies that support the management of their illness, or rather management of themselves as someone who is ill. Becoming absorbed with an activity can bring us into the present moment and into a place less overshadowed by illness and where, for a short time, life might appear more expansive. Often people who have enjoyed art-making want to do the same kind of thing at home.

The 'making conscious' nature of the work depends to some extent on the degree of insight the person has about their situation, although a person can be deeply involved without wanting to articulate why. The activity can be simple or sophisticated: making, playing, in the context of a relationship with the artist.

What is created always communicates something of the person and what they think and feel about what is happening to them. The feelings evoked in the artist about the patient are also important guides. The artist is a witness, acknowledging and validating, being a mirror, reflecting to the person they are working with a sense of themselves.

Meetings do, and should, vary in length. The variation depends on the patient's energy levels and the state of their health. A patient may be very ill yet a short time of doodling or humming might be of great significance. It can take place in the person's home, often at the bedside. It may involve other members of the family which changes the nature of the work that we do, and sometimes this is very positive and sometimes not. One can get to know the patient in their family relationships and dynamics and witness both the positive and the negative aspects of this. Sometimes it is important to persist in organising a private session for the patient in his own home. You may have a designated art room where you work, and also have access to other rooms that are shared with other staff. You might want to work with a person in the garden, or another public space. All are right and we need to be guided by the people we work with and what is both possible and expected by them.

I always keep my own process notes of sessions and I also contribute to the patient's multi-disciplinary notes. I keep the work created safely, but, in reality, most people take what they have made home with them. Often, with their permission, we exhibit or perform the work together.

Case study: 'B.' – making a relationship through painting and music

I want to describe the series of individual sessions I had with B. to illustrate the importance of expecting the unexpected, and of needing a flexible artistic response. She was an elderly lady with cancer and a patient on the hospice inpatient unit. She previously attended the Anniversary Centre, initially as an outpatient, although I had never worked with her in any of the art groups which I ran there. She regularly came down from the inpatient unit to the Anniversary Centre in her bed. She was referred to myself as a community artist, the reason being given that she had become more frustrated by her communication difficulties brought on by her illness and that she might benefit from some input. I met her one day in the Anniversary Centre where I discovered that she was confined to her bed and quite restless and uncomfortable. While she was pleased to meet me and talk briefly about where she had lived and the work she had done in retail, it was clear that her communication skills were affected by her brain tumour and she was frustrated when she could not correctly name certain things. Her speech was sometimes unintelligible. Overall she was restless and after some unsatisfactory adjusting of pillows she asked me if I would comb her hair. I found her comb and began to comb her hair. Her agitation subsided a little. I spent our first session combing her hair and just sitting with her. At the end of the session she said she felt dreadful. She indicated she would like me to visit her on the ward, or maybe bring her down to the art studio in her bed so that we could perhaps paint.

For our next session, we brought B. down to the art studio in her bed as requested. B. used a paintbrush to put paint to paper and I helped her by steadying her hand. The act of both of us focussing on the same action seemed to make our communication more concrete. Through verbally responding to the marks she made I was also able to establish that she was painting yellow flowers in a fondly-remembered garden. We continued to bring B. to the art studio in her bed but in the subsequent two sessions she declined to paint and asked me to paint for her. At first I did not think this was a good idea but reluctantly agreed. She was clear about the colours she wanted and in retrospect I realise that she was 'dictating' the images to me in order to make them a reality. Our conversation focussed more and more on her feeling fed up of being ill and wanting to die. The images that emerged from her instructions and my interpretations mirrored this conversation. One painting was a dark veiled female figure that could also have been a doorway, and another was a group of flying fish swimming upwards through the sea and into the air. Although I was uncomfortable with painting 'for' her, it was of some importance to her as she was so insistent. She also continued to express her desire for her life to be over.

In one of our sessions she was too restless to give painting instructions to me and while being made comfortable by one of the nurses who helped us bring her bed down to the arts studio, she asked the nurse to sing for her. The nurse declined but I said I would be happy to and B. and I sang 'Daisy, Daisy', 'You Are My Sunshine', and 'A Nightingale Sang in Berkeley Square' together.

The following meeting we had was to be our last. Due to the singing in the previous session, I decided to play the guitar for her and this led to a markedly different experience. As I played the guitar she lay back among her pillows and relaxed, which was unusual. B. sometimes mouthed the words of the song I was singing but mostly she listened with an uncommon, profound stillness. There appeared to be no struggle and she appeared content and at peace.

I learned that she died the following week. Although the sessions with B. were characterised by difficulties in communicating, it was clear to me that she was able to make a relationship with painting and music which enabled her to have a different and new experience of herself together with another human being.

Working with groups

I work with groups of people on a weekly basis who attend the Anniversary Centre (the day and outpatient centre at St Christopher's), and in a variety of local care homes. Sometimes we are joined by family members and carers, or in-patients from the wards. We also mirror these groups in other community venues, such as care homes. With the other artists who I work alongside, we each run the group for an eight-week period. The art form to be used is usually chosen by the artist drawing on their own arts background and the theme is offered and discussed and agreed by the attendees at the group.

There is normally a consultation between artist and the nursing staff in order to assess each patient's needs, their interests, and their progress in the group is monitored through daily meetings and the weekly multi-disciplinary meetings. Attendees at each of the groups are invited to explore a variety of arts media: painting, drawing, printing, ceramics, photography, music-making, song-writing, other kinds of creative writing and life-story work. A theme is often suggested to focus and stimulate the group's creativity – 'Personal landscapes', 'Musical landmarks in my life,' 'Painting myself', and so on.

The exploration is offered as a journey to be enjoyed, an opportunity to play, often to try something new and to be surprised. The group may connect with and express some of their creative vitality, the fullness of their individual and group personality not only defined by the term 'patient' or 'ill person'. It is also offered as a challenge, as another way of focussing on what is happening to them. The group can become a place where being with other patients brings encouragement, understanding and the freedom to share. People living with similar realities can feel less isolated and more supported. There is the potential for honest exchanges, for becoming more comfortable with being vulnerable, being more comfortable and accepting about crying and being angry.

These groups can also be used as places to hide and to pretend, to form cliques, and to project difficult feelings; places of sabotage, of tension, of denial and of scapegoating. After all, when groups come together, real life is always portrayed, and just because someone is dying, this does not make them a saint. Some people attending the groups may not have many group skills or have lost the confidence in social interaction through their illness and isolation.

So my aim is simply for the group to be a group, each person bringing all of who they are and supporting them to find the courage to talk about difficulties and fears, to break taboos around talking about death and what it means to be dying, to find strength and to be seen and to be heard. The person who chooses only to observe is also a participant.

In reality the membership of the group is constantly changing; sporadic attendance through illness, hospital appointments, disease progression, death, the temporariness of inpatient attendance. I find this challenging because it reinforces a sense of not being in control. However, I have learned that such situations demand flexibility and I have to adapt to how it is rather than wondering what it might be. I could be thinking all of the week about how the work with someone might be developing and then they are absent. In spite of this, groups form and patients enjoy the work. They become attached both to the group and to each other and enjoy the work.

Case study: sharing stories between patients and school children

I want to relate my recent experience of running a group for patients which involved a group of students from the Brit School in Croydon. We have run the St Christopher's Schools Project with local primary, secondary, special schools and colleges since 2004. There is an information and guidance pack which is available from the St Christopher's website, which gives advice and examples of how this project works (see www.stchristophers. org.uk). The project has been a real success, with other hospices across the UK and other organisations across the world picking up the project idea and creating their own versions of it. Much has been written about its execution and success (Hartley and Payne 2008).

We always follow a simple, structured format. After meeting students in school and explaining what the hospice is and what it does, and encouraging students to ask questions and share expectations, we organise four sessions on site with patients. We usually propose an art or music-based theme so that patients and students can engage with something that has an end product which, in turn, can help them to engage with each other. The arts give a context for these two opposing groups to come together. The first session is a meeting and an introduction. Two sessions of using the creative arts together follow, and the project concludes with a celebration which includes an exhibition or a performance of the work which has been created as part of the project. The aim of the project is to simply change attitudes towards the hospice, death and dying, as well as offering dying patients and their family members an opportunity to remain part of normal life.

The Brit School specialises in the performing arts and technology. The 16–17-year-olds who joined this project were specialising in music and drama and they were invited to get to know a group of patients with an age range of between 40–95. Through a series of games and exercises they shared their likes and dislikes. This led to listening to patients' life stories including such things as descriptions of what it was like to discover that you had been diagnosed with a life-threatening illness. With the patients' permission the students went away and worked on the stories they had been told, returning the following week with songs, poems and re-enactments of scenes from patients' lives. In the final week the students presented a performance of this work in the Anniversary Centre, having shown it beforehand to patients for approvable, criticism and direction. A parting gift to each patient was a CD of a powerful song that the students had written together and recorded along with excerpts of dialogue which had been recorded as part of the project, giving both students and patients the opportunity to share their thoughts on the subjects of illness and death.

Initially it was difficult to see how the project would work as on the first meeting the group of teenagers sat or stood awkwardly in front of the group of patients of many different ages, united only by the fact of being terminally ill. But the photographic record of all of the meetings captures the quality of contact between patients, family members and students, the steady gazes, the laughter and the tears. Some patients shared their pride at the way their stories were given back to them as the project developed. Individual students shared how their experience of patients living courageously with dying caused them to look at their own lives in a more meaningful way. They said that young people did not necessarily value life, and here were people valuing every moment that they had left. The frank and honest sharing by patients about their fear and grief and their loss of health was sometimes hard for the students to listen to, but each week the atmosphere of mutual respect and encouragement grew even stronger. I could see that many people were profoundly touched by their encounters. I was also struck by how quickly the two groups began to share their experiences openly together. I think the project worked well in the Anniversary Centre day and outpatient setting because it is fundamentally a meeting place, where social encounters can be supported and developed. The concluding performance was held in this centre, a public space at the heart of the hospice where patients, family members, carers, other visitors, staff, volunteers and students and their family members could gather together. The performance was both light and serious, celebratory and at times often quite painful to be part of. The audience was moved, particularly by the range of feelings expressed, the maturity of this expression and also by the way people's lives were honoured.

Exhibitions and performances

Exhibitions and performances of artwork created with patients and families are an important part of the artistic process (Hartley and Payne 2008). It is unusual for art which is created by artists to be private and never seen, so it is important that we always give this option to the people who we work with who are coming to the end of their lives. Naturally I talk with people about the work they produce and the process they have gone through to make it, with the view towards an exhibition or performance. The question of audience is important to take into account. Sometimes, of course, the work is intended for friends and family members as gifts and legacies or as signs that they are still creative and alive. In my experience, most people are happy to show, speak, play, or sing their work to a wider audience. Something they are pleased with and proud of can be acknowledged, affirmed and applauded. It can also continue to grow in significance for them and others. Thus it is good, in my experience, to show the work to others – particularly in a group situation – because the response is invariably positive and because allowing our artwork to be seen or to be heard by others can freshen our own perspective, helping us to take ourselves more seriously. Exhibiting the work can also develop things further, bringing enrichment to oneself and to a wider audience. Exhibitions and performances can also empower the author and inspire them to further explore themselves as an artist. Organising a musical performance or a poetry reading can be moving, enriching and affirming. As part of the work I do, organising exhibitions and performances is very important. They provoke a wide range of responses and reactions and are a sign of liveliness and, above all, they celebrate people's lives.

Exhibitions at the hospice also give a reason to invite in groups of people who might normally not come into such a building. Viewing the hospice as an 'art gallery' or 'performance venue' can help change people's view both of the hospice and the work that is done there. Viewing artwork, or listening to performances created by people who are living with death on a daily basis, can also give the exhibition experience a different sense of reality. I find that members of the local community who view the exhibitions are deeply moved by their experience and consequently form healthier connections with the hospice and those who use its services. We also hold regular exhibitions and performances of work created at the hospice in other community venues such as doctors' surgeries, local libraries and art galleries. These also provide opportunities for taking the work of the hospice and the importance of the arts in such settings out to a wider audience.

Reflection

Mick shares with us his very personal motivation for coming to work as a community artist in end of life care. He tells us of some of the challenges which day and outpatient care within hospices raises and faces within the health and social care environment. As part of reflecting on Mick's work, I would like to outline the development of the Anniversary Centre, a new centre for providing day and outpatient services at St Christopher's Hospice. As already mentioned, hospice day care centres have undergone a critical examination over the past years and a number of inefficacies and challenges have been highlighted. The Anniversary Centre has been one way of addressing these challenges.

The Anniversary Centre opened at the end of July 2009. It was made possible both by a £2.5 million capital appeal, and some detailed development work around the challenges facing specialist palliative day care and outpatient services.

As mentioned earlier, many of the problems and challenges facing hospice day care were emphasised during research studies carried out between 2000 and 2005 (Douglas *et al.* 2000, 2003, 2005). Important issues were highlighted around equity of access, patients' preferences, the high costs of running services, and whether attendance at day care affected the use of other specialist palliative care services. The findings concluded that there was no evidence to justify day care on grounds of health economics, quality of life or symptom control. Most groups of day care users did not represent the cultural mix of the wider communities within which they lived, and attendance at day care did not guarantee a more effective use of other health and social care services. It is worth mentioning that our own research at St Christopher's highlighted some of the more positive themes which Douglas *et al.* had identified as part of their research, namely that people benefitted from meeting others who were 'in the same boat'. The social aspects of coming together with others were highlighted as being very beneficial. Other issues also came up as important such as that of nurses being important in order to make their visit to the hospice 'feel secure'.

A number of focus planning groups were held with users of our services to assist with project planning. The following core themes emerged:

1. *More flexible timing:* Many patients did not want to restrict attendance between 10am and 3pm. For example, they might prefer to arrive at 1pm and stay until 6pm.

2. *One-stop-shop:* It was common that people wanted to sort out their problems in one visit. For example, to have a series of co-ordinated appointments to see the nurse, physiotherapist and social worker.

3. *Not always coming alone:* Some felt it was important for them to bring family members and friends.

4. *Bathing service:* Many patients wanted to be able to book a bath, in order to bath themselves with help at hand if needed as they were too anxious to bath at home in case something went wrong.

The new vision was to address the common themes raised in the focus groups, while also concentrating on the challenges highlighted as part of the research studies. We were also clear that the new centre should only require minimal additional resource in terms of staffing, hence the development of the new volunteer training programme mentioned later in this chapter.

The centre is open seven days a week between 8am and 9pm, and provides:

- a large social space for all St Christopher's users (including those attending for planned day care)

- an information area with internet access

- a café with a 'healthy food' menu

- a bathing suite

- a rehabilitation gym

- areas for relaxation and spiritual contemplation

- access to a range of group work possibilities

- access to a range of clinic and therapy appointments.

Planned day care, which is run by a small nursing team, takes place Monday to Friday with plans to offer new possibilities at the weekend in the near future. People can come and go as they please, as long as they catch up with their specialist nurse.

The social space also offers the option for users to 'drop-in' at any time in order to search for information or enjoy some refreshments in the café.

Patients attending a planned group activity, such as circuit training, pilates and fatigue and breathlessness management in the rehabilitation gym, or creative arts programmes and finance management groups, together with those waiting for a range of clinic appointments, for example with the doctor, community nurse specialist or complementary therapist, also use the space. It is also available for families and inpatients, bereaved people, or those coming to view a body in our viewing rooms. It has been surprising how this eclectic mix of people collectively affected by a range of end of life issues instinctively come together to offer each other mutual, healthy support.

The strap line *'You come to us when you are able, and we'll come to you when you're not'* offers a new drive to encourage those patients and families who are able to come and see their community nurse specialist and other health care professionals in a clinic setting and have their care managed on site. We all know that for some, attending the hospice day centre is the last thing they can imagine or want. We believe that for some of these people, following an initial CNS assessment in the home, this opportunity will enable them to see what else is available in the centre as listed above. Following their clinic appointment, they may decide to attend a group, use the gym or information facilities, or just stay for lunch.

It is important to mention that volunteers are key to the success of the new Anniversary Centre. Mick mentions the challenges of training volunteers and addressing this has been very important. A 12-week training programme furnishes them with the skills needed to provide hospitality and a 'listening ear' as well as to signpost users to the most appropriate information they need. They are also given a working knowledge of the multi-disciplinary team as well as mandatory training such as moving and handling and food handling. Their commitment enables us to keep the centre open later into the evening and over the weekend.

We believe it is important to keep our users motivated and independent as long as possible. Therefore, all patients and carers attending the centre are asked to make their own way in. As a back-up to this, we employ a full-time minibus driver who will pick people up when they are not able to get themselves in. At present, 44 per cent of people make their own way into planned day care, as opposed to 9 per cent before the centre opened.

During the time since the centre opened, the number of people attending for a planned day has risen considerably. In addition to this, the number of people coming through the centre on a daily basis has averaged between 150 and 200. Although there is still a lot more work to be done with regard to achieving our vision and aims, we believe that the Anniversary Centre at St Christopher's is beginning to offer a more useful and cost effective range of day and outpatient services to our users in a more appropriate and flexible way.

With regard to continuing to develop the new centre, one of the issues that we are focussing on is to change the way that the hospice, death and dying is viewed across society. It is clear that one of the major failings of the hospice movement and the development of such services across the world has been the failure to change general public attitudes towards the end of life. Most people would still rather not talk about it, and for many, the thought of visiting a hospice can be terrifying. In 2009, the National Council for Palliative Care established the 'Dying Matters' coalition with the aim of bringing together a broad range of groups and organisations across the UK in order to work together so that death and dying might be more firmly planted within the national psyche. This agency works on a national level through major campaigning and developing a range of tools and systems for both professionals and members of the public to use in order to navigate their way through important issues. People can discover how to make a will, or plan a funeral, or learn skills on how to open up conversations with friends or family members about wishes and needs regarding the end of life. For many hospices, as well as providing good end of life care, promoting the work that they do has always been important. An initiative at St Christopher's has been to open the Anniversary Centre to the general public as well as to patients, family members and friends. A social programme offers regular, planned events such as a professional concert series, a Sunday lunch menu with live music, a weekly curry night, a pizza night, a community choir and a quilting group, in order to bring together users of services with members of the general public. A recent successful initiative 'Death Chat at St Christopher's' brings groups of people together over cheese and wine to discuss issues around death and dying more directly. The message is that dying is a normal activity, and in many circumstances, can be managed well. This new programme has been very successful in engaging the local community within the actual work of the hospice on a day to day basis. Although it has been created to change the attitudes of the general public towards the work of the hospice, in many ways it also gives patients and families who are using the hospice services a sense of still being 'normal' and not being segregated from the community they live in just because they are facing death.

Like St Christopher's, many other hospices across the UK have developed new day and outpatient services in order to respond to the challenges of providing end of life care to more people at less cost.

It is more likely now that day care centres market themselves as 'one-stop-shops', where people can access a range of services in one setting, as information centres which are not only open to those people in the last months of their life, but open to a broader selection of people, as cafés with internet access where patients, families and members of the public can come and go as they please.

It remains to be seen whether this kind of response can offer a more successful, suitable and cost effective way for a greater number of people to access end of life care services and information in the way they need to, when they need to, whoever they happen to be.

References

Clark, D. (2002) *Cicely Saunders: Founder of the Hospice Movement. Selected Letters 1959–1999.* Oxford: Oxford University Press.

Copp, G., Richardson, A., McDaid, P. and Marshall Searson, D.A. (1998) 'A telephone survey of the provision of palliative day care services.' *Palliative Medicine 12*, 161–170.

Douglas, H.R., Higginson, I.J., Myers, K. and Normand, C.E. (2000) 'Assessing structure, process and outcome in palliative day care: A pilot study for a multi-centre trail.' *Health and Social Care in the Community 8*, 5, 336–344.

Douglas, H.R., Normand, C.E., Higginson, I.J. and Goodwin, D.M. (2005) 'A new approach to eliciting patients' preferences for palliative day care: The choices experiment method.' *Journal of Pain and Symptom Management 29*, 5, 435–445.

Douglas, H.R., Normand, C.E., Higginson, I.J., Goodwin, D.M. and Myers, K. (2003) 'Palliative day care: What does it cost to run a centre and does attendance affect the use of other services?' *Palliative Medicine 17*, 628–637.

Doyle, D. (2002) *Volunteers in Hospice and Palliative Care – A Handbook for Volunteer Service Managers.* Oxford: Oxford University Press.

Fisher, R. and McDaid, P. (1996) *Palliative Day Care.* London: Edward Arnold.

Hartley, N. and, Payne, M. (2008) *The Creative Arts in Palliative Care.* London and Philadelphia, PA: Jessica Kingsley Publishers.

Hearn, J. and Myers, K. (2001) *Palliative Day Care in Practice.* Oxford: Oxford University Press.

Chapter 7

Working in Community Settings

Gerry Prince and Nigel Hartley

Introduction

During this chapter, we pick up on, and explore, some essential points to be considered when working with people within the places that they live. Within the central part of the chapter, we hear from Gerry, who works as a musician and a music therapist. Following some information regarding Gerry's background, we hear about some of the key points to be considered when working in a variety of community venues, including people's own homes. These are headed as follows:

- The home environment

- Referral procedures

- Lone working and personal safety

- Working with someone within their home

- Community nurse specialists as key links and mentors

- Useful instruments and materials to transport and use

- Travelling in the community

- Supporting people living with dementia and an introduction to the National Dementia Strategy

- The practicalities of providing services into care homes

- Differences between working with children and adults

- Supporting funerals.

Some short stories are added into the mix to guide us through. I end the chapter with a short reflection.

Gerry: my background

My name is Gerry Prince and I started playing piano as a child but switched to DJ-ing in my teens before learning to play bass and joining a band in my early 20s. The next two decades were spent playing bass guitar and keyboards in my own and other people's bands and recording in studios as a session musician and songwriter. I also worked as a programmer and producer in the commercial music industry. During this time, I was lucky enough to work with a diverse range of artists from the Senegalese singer Baaba Maal to the Bristol Hip Hop group, Massive Attack.

I first encountered music therapy while studying for a music degree in 2000 at City University London; the module was to change the course of my life. I decided that this was a profession I wished to be part of. When a few years later, I joined the Nordoff-Robbins Master's music therapy training course with a view to working within special needs education, I never imagined that this path would lead to working in end of life care at St Christopher's Hospice.

I first came to St Christopher's in the second year of the course as a student on placement. I knew little of hospices prior to the placement other than that they cared for terminally ill patients. The only reference to them in my life had been the death of a flatmate's father in a Midlands hospice. She spoke of the staff in glowing terms and of how they had helped to make the unbearable bearable. During the placement I spent a term working alongside a multi-disciplinary team including nurses, physiotherapists, spiritual care workers, occupational therapists and a team of artists, all responsible for the care and wellbeing of adults over the age of 18 who were facing the end of their lives, and their families. It was a challenging placement but an experience I valued, so when St Christopher's advertised a post for a music therapist shortly after I had completed my course, I applied for the job and was successful. I have now worked part-time at the hospice for over five years.

What makes the hospice a unique place to work at is that I am part of a unique team comprising music and other arts therapists, community musicians and artists. We each bring a diversity of life experience, training and different perspectives to our work together with our own individual strengths and weaknesses. In my experience, this mix creates and supports a refreshing and healthy atmosphere to work in and also challenges and prevents polarisation of attitudes. It also affords opportunities for giving and receiving a lot of support in a challenging field of work.

I am going to focus on much of the work which I have been involved in providing within people's homes, including care homes.

The home environment

Working with patients in their own homes provides an opportunity to discover important aspects of their life that a visit from them to the hospice does not. Some of the questions that I find useful to ask myself when I first visit someone at home are:

- How does the patient live their life?

- What kind of contact does the patient have with the outside world?

- How involved are any family members or friends and what kind of support mechanism do they provide for the patient?

Objects around the home, as well as being useful triggers for conversation, can also inform us about the patient's life, both past and present, and also their interests. These might include:

- photographs of the patient, together with family and friends

- collections of certain objects

- paintings and other artworks hung on the walls

- music which is playing on the radio or CD player, or music which people listen to on an iPod

- musical instruments or art materials around the home.

All of these enable a picture to be built up of how the person lives and copes with their illness and also informs us about, and feeds into, the context within which our work will take place. I occasionally have to deal with extraneous noise from televisions, radios and sometimes negotiate that they are turned off during the time I am together with someone at home.

Case study: extraneous noise

The wife of a patient acutely aware of her husband's discomfort and need for privacy in his music sessions would leave the house for the duration of our sessions. Before she left, she would make sure that both the radio and the television were switched off.

Referral procedures

A referral is normally picked up at the hospice and will come from another member of the multi-disciplinary team, usually the community nurse specialist. Sometimes I will have been working with the person when they have been to the hospice either as a day patient or outpatient. This might have either been on a one to one basis, or, more than likely, as part of a group. Their illness may have deteriorated and we will have decided to continue working together within the person's home. I normally telephone the person to make an appointment and this is particularly important if I have not met the person before.

Before setting out on a home visit, I have found it to be an imperative to read the most recent additions to the patient's notes, as well as to talk to any other professionals who have recently visited the person at home. Sometimes I might learn that the person is less well, has been admitted to hospital, or that they have died.

Lone working and personal safety

As an artist or arts therapist working in a palliative care setting you should, at some point, find yourself out in the community visiting patients who are too unwell to come into the hospice. After all, most care given by hospices is given within the home and not within the hospice building. St Christopher's looks after around 850 people within their own homes on any one day, with 48 inpatient beds to support this work within the hospice building (see www.stchristophers.org.uk). As well as working within people's own homes, I have also found that I am expected to do outreach work within other institutions such as other hospices, care homes and schools. I have learned that important advice to keep in mind regarding home visits include:

- Read the patient's multi-disciplinary notes before embarking on a visit.

- Look for important information regarding the patient's history of illness, visits by other health care professionals, risk assessments of falls and infection, etc. It might be important to know if the person has animals, or if there is any possible risk of violence from the patient or family members. This kind of information will be listed in the multi-disciplinary notes.

- Talk to the patient's community nurse specialist and/or other colleagues at the hospice to get first-hand information about the patient and the home environment. Sometimes things change very quickly with patients, so I always find it essential to keep right up to date.

- Read the lone worker policy, which outlines the procedures to be adhered to while undertaking a home visit.

The lone worker policy will list vital steps to take such as informing other members of your team or line manager about the date, time and length of the visit (see Table 7.1.) I let my colleagues know the likely time that the visit will finish and arrange to telephone when I am expecting to return from the visit and address of where I will be; I also always check if the person is able to answer the door when I arrive, or if someone will be present to answer the door. There may well be a 'key safe' (a small box at the front door which houses the key for the property). If this is the case, I need to make sure that I have the combination to be able to open it and access the key to enter the person's home.

Case study: safety issues on home visits

I recently made a home visit to a patient who was a musician. The flat he lived in looked like a tornado had passed through it but of greater concern was the fact that he had overloaded all his plug sockets. I wanted to record the session but my assessment of the situation was, while it felt safe to be in the room, plugging anything into his electrical supply was unadvisable. I recorded the session but on a battery-operated system and also spoke with him about the dangers of overloading the sockets and helped him find someone who would come into his flat and advise him on how best to use his electronic equipment.

Table 7.1: An example of lone working guidelines

Procedures for Therapists, etc. Undertaking Home Visits
When any of the professional groups above do a home visit alone the following should apply:
• They should carry their own charged mobile phone which must be switched on.

• They should inform the relevant person:
  ◦ The name, address and phone number of the person being visited.
  ◦ The type, colour and registration number of the car they are using.
  ◦ The number of the mobile phone they are carrying.
  ◦ When they expect to return to the hospice.

• These details should be written in the home visits appointment book which is with the relevant person.
• In the absence of the relevant person, or if their visit is expected to conclude after 5pm, they should inform the receptionist on duty.
• On return to the hospice they should immediately inform their contact.
• If they foresee that they will be later than expected in returning from the visit they should telephone their contact to let them know.
• If the target time for return has passed, the following sequence should be carried out:
Check if a message has been left with relevant area. If no message:
1. Phone the office of the member of staff to see if message has been left. If no message
2. Phone the member of staff making the visit. If no reply
3. Contact the patient. If no reply
4. Phone the member of staff making the visit on their home number. If no reply
5. Discuss with the senior manager re: next decision.
6. Phone the police.
• If a response is obtained from the member of staff making the visit but it is suspected that they are under duress, go straight to action (Lone Working Review, April 2013).
• If the member of staff making the visit calls their office and informs a colleague of change of a plan, the colleague must let the relevant person know.

Working with someone within their home

When I first meet a person within their own home, I have noticed that they may sometimes be a little guarded as I have only spoken to them previously on the telephone. My experience has shown that they might be concerned about what I might be demanding of them. After all, an artist or arts therapist visiting someone at home is, for many people, out of the ordinary. People expect to be visited at home by doctors, nurses and a range of other health care professionals, but artists are somewhat unexpected.

The fact that I am a guest in a person's home environment affects how I behave and, in turn, affects how they behave. The dynamic will be different from seeing someone in the hospice building. I have discovered that the person is more likely to feel at ease and less on their guard than they might do within an institutional setting. It is also important to realise that an ill person will have visits at home from many health care professionals during their week and that I am one of many. I sometimes experience that the person I am visiting may also be concerned that they are being judged, especially if their home is chaotic and not in what they feel to be a presentable state.

Case study: embarrassment about home visits

One patient I had previously worked with in the hospice and established a good relationship with steadfastly refused home visits when her condition worsened despite a keen interest and understanding of the value of engaging with the arts and how they related to her wellbeing. She was too embarrassed by the chaotic state her house had fallen into as a consequence of her illness.

I have found it common that family members often use the opportunity when I am visiting to offload their problems, feelings or fears. Whenever I feel that the family member or carer needs support for themselves, I find it important to feed this back to the multi-disciplinary team.

I occasionally find myself facing the situation where a family member or the patient wishes me to leave earlier or stay longer than I have planned. It is always important to be as flexible as possible with time, in order to respond to unexpected issues which might arise.

I have often experienced, when I arrive at someone's home, that there is a feeling of the person not wishing me to be there. There is the possibility that once organised, the patient might feel pressurised to have the session even if, when I arrive, they may not wish to do so. They might be aware of the distance I have travelled and might feel guilty about cancelling our meeting at that point, whereas in the hospice a client may feel more comfortable about cancelling a session if they are not feeling up to it.

Case study: how well the patient may be feeling

I was working with a patient in his home. The sessions were going well. However, on one visit (I had previously telephoned to confirm) I detected an unwillingness to participate in the session. This dissipated as the session went on but I remarked about it to him and he admitted that between my phone call and my arrival he had felt less well and had wanted to cancel. He was, however, glad he had not done so as improvising music with me had lifted his mood.

Community nurse specialists as key links and mentors

As well as offering support and guidance regarding pain and symptom management, the community nurse specialist (CNS) provides patients with psychosocial support and helps with welfare issues, spiritual care and organising carer support. They are the patient's link to the other professional teams at the hospice (including the artists/arts therapists) as well as outside agencies within the community (see www.stchristophers.org.uk). As such they are the key contact point when organising home visits and are likely to be the instigators of referrals to the artist or arts therapist for the patient as part of their initial assessment, or they may organise a referral responding to a patient's request.

The CNS is an invaluable source of information and can provide feedback regarding your work that a patient may be unable or unwilling to give to you face to face.

Case study: useful feedback from a CNS

Working with a patient who suffered dysphasia I was able to monitor the progress of his therapy through reports from his CNS who was around to see the impact of the work following each of the meetings I had. This feedback was invaluable regarding the on-going work and enabled me to plan accordingly.

The CNS will also be aware of familial dynamics that may be affecting the patient and which might manifest themselves in your meetings within the home. They will know of the other interventions and work of different professionals and the impact that these may be having on the patient, and can pass on information regarding any changes in a patient's condition and circumstances, and also advise on practical issues such as moving and handling or on the patient's motor skills. While this information may well be available in the patient's notes, I have found that they can furnish me with other information that the notes might not provide based on their on-going relationship with the patient.

Case studies: practical support and overview from a CNS

A music therapist, making home visits to a patient who had difficulty swallowing but would request water during the music session, was supported by the patient's CNS who taught the therapist the correct procedure necessary to assist the patient to drink safely.

Also, when an arts therapist became aware that the patient they were visiting was giving them very different information than they were giving to other health care professionals who were also visiting, consulting the patient's CNS enabled the team to gain a more rounded picture of the patient's experience. This, in turn, helped the professionals concerned work more successfully together on behalf of the patient.

Developing good working relationships with the CNS by discussing the work being done helps both the on-going work with the patient and, in turn, may lead to more appropriate referrals. The better the CNS understands the how and why of the arts-working process, the greater the possibility to make appropriate referrals.

Useful instruments and materials
to transport and use

As a music therapist or community musician the type of instruments that can usefully be transported will be determined by the context you are planning to be working in. With patients on home visits I like to cover harmonic, sonic and melodic possibilities that give the patient a variety of musical experiences but are light and portable. I usually take with me:

- a small hand harp

- a pentatonic thumb piano

- a small metallophone

- a tambourine

- a small hand drum

- a portable recording device

- a range of beaters

- a guitar.

These are the instruments I can transport either in the car, on the bus or train, or on my bicycle. Sometimes you might think that if you are using a car you can take more and larger instruments, however, you cannot rely on the fact that you will be able to park near the house, and may need to walk a long way. When working in institutions such as care homes or other hospices where I run groups, I normally take a bag holding a variety of smaller percussion instruments and a guitar.

The community artists and arts therapists I work with carry a small selection of materials on home visits, including:

- watercolours

- pencils

- pastels

- a selection of brushes

- an eraser

- a pencil sharpener

- a roll of paper or an art pad

- a piece of board which can be used as a resting board to work on.

These can all be normally carried in a soft holdall.

Travelling in the community

Working in the patient's home, or within other organisations in the hospice catchment area should be part and parcel of our everyday work and of providing a comprehensive arts service. I have experienced that good planning is vital in order to work as effectively as possible when working outside of the hospice building. Initial questions which I always ask myself include:

- How many visits am I expecting to make in the day?

- How does this affect my other commitments within the institution?

If I am travelling by car, I plan a route beforehand and ensure that parking will not be an issue. I make sure to leave enough time to carry out the journey and add on a bit of extra time in case there are any hold-ups. If I am travelling by public transport, I decide geographically who it makes sense to visit first and whether I need to make more than one appointment. I keep any travel tickets in order to claim any expenses incurred.

Through experience I have learned to make a point of telephoning the person I am visiting beforehand in order to confirm the meeting is still going ahead and to let them know that I am on my way. I also always carry a small geographical 'A–Z' as a safety measure.

Supporting people living with dementia and an introduction to the National Dementia Strategy

We are told that people are living longer. One reason for this will be current developments in health care and the resulting more effective drug treatment programmes (Pace, Treloar and Scott 2011).

The increase in the number of older people living longer will also result in an increase in the number of people living with dementia. As a consequence, we are also told that more older people will die in care homes from multiple chronic illnesses that will include dementia (Bern-Klug 2010).

Case study: the Keeping Relationships Alive project

One of our recent restricted funding projects called 'Keeping Relationships Alive', funded by the St James' Place Foundation, focussed on the use of music with people who were living with dementia in care homes. We ran a series of workshops and groups over a period of two years in a number of care homes across South East London. Our intention was to give care home residents a new experience of themselves through musical activity, but also to teach care home staff simple skills to equip them to use music with residents, and show them how this experience could give them a new experience of the residents that they care for. The project was successful and we felt that we learned a lot, including how music can reach the most isolated and vulnerable people and enable them to step out of their frailty and isolation into a more active and dynamic set of relationships. We also learned how important it is for us to be able to give away our knowledge and equip care home staff, who sometimes can feel isolated and unsupported, to do something practical and purposeful, thus giving them more self-confidence.

In recent years, there has been a cultural shift in the perspective of the care requirements of dementia patients at the end of life and a subsequent paradigm shift in how dementia is viewed (Bern-Klug 2010).

Moves have been taken to improve the quality of care provided to end of life patients in care home settings through the introduction of palliative care services and palliative care approaches (Bern-Klug 2010).

As a music therapist working in a palliative care setting I have experienced this development through my involvement in the hospice's care home nursing team, who have been working to embed the Gold Standards Framework (GSF) into local care homes (Hansford and Meeham 2007).

Although the illness does not have the clear stages of cancer disease progression, it is clear that people with dementia may exhibit symptoms which might include:

- depression
- loss of mobility
- inability to communicate verbally
- problems with swallowing
- incontinence
- weight loss.

These symptoms may not be present simultaneously but their presence is indicative of a patient at the end stage of life (NHS 2012).

Dementia, a degenerative neurological disease, currently affects approximately 700,000 individuals across the UK. The majority of people who live with dementia are aged over 65 but there is a sizeable minority living with the disease under this age (Alzheimer's Society 2012). With an expected increase in the number of people living with dementia and the increasing cost of caring for older people, the first Department of Health National Dementia Strategy – 'Living Well with Dementia' – was published in 2009 responding to the demand for a cohesive policy that takes into account the needs of an ageing population (DH 2009).

The strategy, drawn up by the Department of Health in collaboration with the Alzheimer's Society, outlines ways in which local authorities and health care providers can provide a better level of care and support for dementia patients and their carers. Set over a five-year framework, it seeks to address three main areas:

1. Improvements in diagnosis at all stages of the disease but with emphasis on early diagnosis.

2. Greater awareness and understanding of dementia.

3. Development of services to meet the needs of patients and their families in order to improve their quality of life.

For more detailed information visit www.dh.gov.uk/dementia.

The practicalities of providing services into care homes

When providing services into care homes I always make contact with the care home manager. My experience of this has been helped enormously through working together with the hospice's care home team, who will always have had experience of the care home before I am asked to visit. It is an increasing imperative that hospices work in partnership with care homes in order to improve the quality of care for people coming to the end of their lives within such organisations. Although getting nursing right within such places is important, we also know that in order to support people to die in the best possible way, quality of life is achieved more effectively when supporting people to tell their story and leave behind a legacy (Hartley and Payne 2008). Therefore, the care home nursing team based at St Christopher's can offer a wealth of important information, and this has both shown and given me an excellent example of working together with others in order to achieve shared aims. I always arrange a meeting with the care home manager through an initial telephone call. It is also useful to ask if there is an activities co-ordinator or someone responsible for groups and events being set up and working within the care home. If so, it is also useful to arrange to meet with them, as they will be influential in the success of what is being offered.

If I am going to be providing one to one work within the care home, it has always been important to make clear the criteria for the work upfront in order to help identify patients suitable to work with.

If I am intending to run a group, I find it useful to ask about the care home population. It is useful to know if the residents are local to the area, or if families live a long way away. When organising groups in care homes I have frequently found that the initial response of the care home staff is to suggest that the more cognitively able patients are the ones who would most benefit from the group activity. In response, I find it useful to gently challenge this assumption by clarifying that all residents are welcome, especially those who are more isolated and rarely interact with others. It is amazing what can happen in the context of an art group activity and how the staff's perception of individuals in their care can change.

As mentioned earlier, sharing our skills with care home staff to continue to utilise the arts when we are not around can also be very useful. From experience, I have found it important to consider that my role is not simply to run a group with residents, but also to be there to support staff to engage those they care for in the arts. I talk to carers about the project, encourage them to become involved and to think about what happens when I am not around. I can always tell when the activities have made a positive impact on staff when they show the confidence to carry on the project when I am not around, thus benefitting the whole care home community and sustaining the effects of what has been achieved.

When I meet to discuss any plans with the manager I always ask to be shown around the home. I find it helpful to enquire about the facilities and materials they have which might be useful. I also check, depending on what we agree to do, whether I need to obtain any formal permission. For example, photographs of group activities may require consent forms signed by residents, carers or staff members. It is always important to clarify where any photographs will be used and to talk about any organisational expectations. If I am running an art group, I always ask whether the finished artwork can be displayed within the care home's communal spaces. I permanently travel with my hospice ID badge and in some cases it has been necessary to give the care home manager a copy of my Criminal Records Bureau (CRB) (now Disclosure and Barring Scheme (DBS)) check.

Case study: community music project

I once put together a short community music project with one care home that involved residents with moderate to severe dementia and a group from the local community that used a pub next to the care home. After learning a set of songs which the residents chose, the residents and locals performed their repertoire to all the residents and their family members in the care home and a week later went to the pub and performed the songs to those people using the bar.

To conclude, once you have organised your activity and spoken to the relevant personnel it is simply a case of making the group happen and recording the process. I find it an imperative to document what I do in some way. This can make sure that what is achieved is captured for the future. The documentation can provide a powerful testimony on the efficacy of the work; it might also contribute to an effective exhibition and should be a part of your good working practice. I sometimes use what is recorded in order to write a case study, to put together a presentation or as the basis of a piece of simple evaluation.

In many cases, it is also important to log the work as part of the care home's patient record system as well as keeping your own notes and records.

Differences between working with children and adults

Working in an adult hospice I have occasionally been asked to work with teenage patients who have been referred on from a children's hospice as part of the transition process, and on a couple of occasions a colleague and I have provided group music therapy for children at a nearby children's hospice in the absence of their regular arts therapist. Fewer children suffer life-threatening illnesses than adults and institutions are not necessarily as large. Consequently there are also fewer children's hospices in the UK, which means children and their carers might have to travel greater distances to reach the hospice buildings (EAPC 2012).

Both the nature of terminal illnesses affecting children and the timeline of the illness progression differs from those of adults: hereditary and extremely rare conditions are more common and leukaemia is the most common form of cancer in children (Carter and Leverton 2011). Children with conditions diagnosed in early childhood may live into early adulthood and beyond (EAPC 2012). Similarly to adult hospices the care given will incorporate the family recognising the role parents, carers and siblings play and the emotional impact this will have on them (Brown and Warr 2007). The fact that some children have conditions that are more long term in nature means developmental transitions that children normally undergo must be factored into the care plan, bringing a further layer of complexity for children's hospice services that will not necessarily feature in an adult hospice (ICPCN 2013).

Partly due to advances in medicine, there are a growing number of young adults with life-limiting conditions who previously would have died during childhood. Transitional care has been identified as a major gap in end of life care (Grinyer 2012).

This is the time when children and younger people might fall through the gap of organised care services. There are a number of initiatives recently set up to look at the issues that this raises (Grinyer 2012). We increasingly see new initiatives set up between adult and children's hospices to address these gaps, as well as new projects run by national organisations such as the Teenage Cancer Trust.

The work done with children in an adult hospice may take the form of post and pre-bereavement sessions and school educational programmes (St Christopher's 2012). Bereavement work with children may involve short-term individual sessions with the child or family with either the dying parent or the surviving parent and will focus on supporting the child through the common issues faced when a parent, or family member is dying (Christ 2000). Working with children and a dying parent or relative can be an important form of legacy work. Positive memories can be created of being with a parent despite the changes that the parent may be undergoing. While the parent is still living, the arts can provide a way of living through 'active' memories as well as developing a legacy to leave behind (Schmidt Peters 2000).

Case study: music to bring a father and son together

A terminally ill mother requested music therapy for herself, her husband and her son with the express aim of helping father and son develop a closer relationship leading up to and after her death. She had been acutely aware of the difficult relationship between her husband and teenage son and saw making and recording music as a way of bringing them together.

Using the arts to bring together school children and hospice patients as part of an educational programme can act as a powerful medium which can change attitudes, both about the work that hospices do and also what it means to be dying. Such programmes form a powerful means of challenging existing stereotypes (St Christopher's 2012).

Supporting funerals

In my experience, the request to be involved in someone's funeral is usually as a result of the relationship that may have developed with the patient and their family during work carried out during the dying process. As a community artist or arts therapist, I am sometimes asked to supply artwork for the funeral which was created as part of my work with the patient, or to provide live music at the funeral. I always feel that it is important to be able to respond to what is needed and attempt to be as straightforward and supportive as possible.

Case study: photographic slideshow at a funeral

A community artist was asked by a patient to take photographs which could be displayed at her funeral. The result was a very moving slideshow displayed during the funeral, which acted as both a focus and a catalyst for people's grief.

Music may feature prominently at funerals (Small 1998). Sometimes I am asked to help to choose hymns or music that the person may wish to have played at their funeral service. Other times I have been asked to provide live music at the event and also to accompany the congregation when singing songs or hymns. As a music therapist or community musician you may well be asked to provide such a service.

I believe it is an important part of my work, and contributes to a sense of bringing work done with the patient and their family to a logical conclusion. At the time of planning and carrying out a funeral, families and friends can be at their most vulnerable. If for any reason I have been unable to help, I try and contact musicians who might be able to carry out the music for the funeral service in order to be of help at a difficult time. For this reason, I find it useful to keep a list of local musicians and local music institutions.

If asked to provide or perform the music at a funeral service, I always maintain good contact with the family leading up to the service. On the day of the service I ensure that I arrive early in order to reassure everyone. I leave plenty of time to make my way to the venue and, if appropriate, I telephone the family to let them know of my arrival. At the place of the service, I find and introduce myself to the person leading the service and inform them of the music I have been asked to perform. I also find it useful to be there early enough to test the acoustics and decide where I will position myself to play from. Finally, I check my instrument and prepare a few words to say about why I am there and my relationship with the dead person in order to put the performance within a meaningful context which can be understood by those attending.

Case study: music as cathartic release

The family of a former young patient requested I play two of the songs I had taught their teenage daughter during music therapy sessions. I had also played these songs at the patient's bedside as she was dying while the family had been present. During the service, when I performed, I became aware of how the songs were acting as a release for much of the grief held by the family and their friends. It was a very cathartic experience and provided an important focus for everyone who attended.

I am sometimes invited to the wake. In my experience, I have always declined as I find that it might provide difficulty both for the family, friends and myself.

Case study: overwhelming experience at a wake

One health care professional told me of time when she had been asked to say a few words at the funeral service of a patient she had supported. When the service had finished she was invited to the wake and she went along. She told me that the family and friends all turned to her for support during the wake, and she realised that her attendance had been misjudged.

Within the context of a hospice, working in the community is an effective way of bringing specialised arts or art therapy services to isolated members of the community and to those unable to visit the hospice itself. This can become a way of ensuring equity of access to all services and a continuity of care which can alleviate, to some degree, anxieties that people may have if they are required, through disease progression, to attend the hospice or become inpatients. Arts therapists and artists working in the community enable the hospice to forge links to other community institutions through community art projects. This helps to enhance the hospice's profile and these projects may provide opportunities both for challenging and changing negative attitudes towards death and dying in a non-threatening and creative manner.

Finally such projects, can be an effective method of sharing specialist arts skills and knowledge with other community workers (for example, care home staff) and in so doing, improve wellbeing and enhance community cohesiveness.

Reflection

Working within a variety of community venues presents us, as professionals, with a specific set of concerns and challenges. What Gerry focusses on throughout his examples is the importance of developing and sustaining relationships with other key professionals in order to make the most cohesive and joined-up experience for, and relationship with, the patient and their family. It is also important, of course, that these relationships, when successfully forged and sustained, can support him to feel that he belongs to something which is much bigger than himself and that he can place the work that he does within a broader, supported context.

Within formal, more therapeutic training programmes, it is unlikely that such issues will have been raised and addressed, and it is unusual for arts therapists to be trained to work within anything other than clearly defined principles of a confidential, boundaried therapeutic relationship. In most cases, this will be defined as expecting to work within a designated therapy room with a person or persons, usually at a repeated time at regular intervals. Many arts therapists are also taught to be reluctant to share the work that they do with a wider group of professionals due to being trained not to break issues of confidentiality. They can easily feel, therefore, that they should not share information which they have learned from the patient as part of their work. However, sharing information between experts in a professional manner can only enhance the work that they all strive to do collectively, and augment the service that the patients and families receive from them.

Something might be learned regarding this from community artists or other practitioners who are likely to be more at ease when working more openly with people within a broad range of different contexts. This will be due to the fact that their professional aim will normally be to create work which can be shared and witnessed more publicly.

What we also experience from Gerry is that many of the assumptions which arts therapists are instilled to expect as part of their work-based experience are promptly challenged when required to work in a variety of less controlled situations and locations. It is clear that training institutions do need to respond to a changing health and social care landscape, where it is demanded that more of the care delivered should take place within people's own homes.

One of the common misconceptions is that the care that hospices offer is delivered within specially designed buildings. It is usual, however, for most hospices that the majority of care given by them will take place within people's own homes, with the hospice building supporting this work with small inpatient units and day care centres. It therefore does not make any sense for any professional not to be providing some of the care that they offer to people within the places that they live. As an example, St Christopher's Hospice provides care at home for around 850 people on any one day, which is supported by a 48-bed inpatient unit and a day and outpatient service. For many hospices, this will be similar, although it is still the case in some instances that some hospices do not provide any home care service, or will be supported to do so by national charitable organisations such as Macmillan. Some other hospice organisations only provide care at home with no inpatient or day care services to back it up.

One of the most useful things we learn from Gerry is that the key to providing a useful arts and art therapy service is to be as flexible and open as possible. Although this does not seem difficult, in reality being able to respond to what is needed, quickly and without fuss, whether the service needs to be delivered within a person's own home, a care home, or other community venue, is an essential part of the artist or arts therapist's developing craft. Keeping the patient and their family central to the process of caring lies at the heart of what good hospice care is all about, providing what people need, whenever they need it, wherever they happen to be. Co-ordinating this care quickly and cost effectively will be crucial if we are to give people the care they require within the location that they require. In order to respond to this complex and demanding task, taking time to contact, converse and share information efficiently with the broad group of professionals involved in a person's end of life care is both sensible and crucial. However, as an artist or arts therapist working part time, this can take a lot of energy and might appear impossible. Gerry, nevertheless, talks of the importance and consequence of good planning and gives some clear examples of how he organises himself as part of his working process, both out of necessity, but also as a professional imperative. It is also clear that he always keeps his work with patients and families central to this process, and as such is able to remain as useful as possible, often under difficult and challenging circumstances.

Working within people's own homes, and other community venues such as care homes, can appear to us to be impossible commissions, especially when such expectations have not been part of any formal training programme. At one moment, we may be travelling to visit a patient at home, at another attempting to contact a different professional involved in the patient's care to share some crucial information, and at another time we might be negotiating our way through some complex funeral arrangements. However, it is important to remember that hospices contain within them a wealth of knowledge and unique experiences, which when sought out and utilised, can motivate, support and guide us to take new steps into uncharted territories.

References

Alzheimer's Society (2012) 'Statistics.' Available at www.alzheimers.org.uk/site/scripts/document_info.php?documentID=341, accessed on 11 June 2013.

Bern-Klug, M. (2010) *Transforming Palliative Care in Care Homes.* New York: Columbia University Press.

Brown, E. and Warr, B. (2007) *Supporting the Child and Family in Paediatric Palliative Care.* London: Jessica Kingsley Publishers.

Carter, B. and Leverton, M. (2004) *Palliative Care for Infants, Children and Adolescents: A Practical Handbook.* Baltimore, MD: Johns Hopkins University Press.

Christ, G.H. (2000) *Healing Children's Grief: Surviving a PArent's Death from Cancer.* New York: Oxford University Press.

DH (Department of Health) (2009) 'Living Well with Dementia: A National Dementia Strategy.' Available at www.gov.uk/government/news/living-well-with-dementia-a-national-dementia-strategy, accessed on 11 June 2013.

EAPC (European Association for Palliative Care) (2012) P*alliative Care for Infants, Children and Young People: The Facts.* Available at www.eapcnet.eu/?TabTd=285, accessed on 1 October 2013.

Grinyer, A. (2012) *Teenage and Young Adult Palliative and End of Life Care Service Evaluation: Home, Hospice and Hospital.* Hoboken, NJ: John Wiley & Sons Ltd.

Hansford, P. and Meeham, H. (2007) *Gold Standards Framework: Improving Community Care.* Available at http://endoflifejournal.stchristophers.org.uk/clinical-practice-development/gold-standards-framework, accessed on 11 June 2013.

Hartley, N. and Payne, M. (2008) *The Creative Arts in Palliative Care.* London and Philadelphia, PA: Jessica Kingsley Publishers.

ICPCN (International Children's Palliative Care Network) (2012) 'What is Children's Palliative Care?' Available at www.icpcn.org.uk/page.asp?section=000100010008004&itemTitle=What+is+Children%92s+Palliative+Care%3F, accessed on 11 June 2013.

NHS (National Health Service) (2012) 'Symptoms of Dementia.' Available at www.nhs.uk/Conditions/dementia-guide/Pages/symptoms-of-dementia.aspx, accessed on 11 June 2013.

Pace, V., Treloar, A. and Scott, S. (2011) *Demetia: From Advanced Disease to Bereavement.* New York: Oxford University Press.

Schmidt Peters, J. (2000) M*usic Therapy: An Introduction. 2nd Edition.* Springfield, IL: Charles Thomas Publisher Ltd.

Small, C. (1998) *Musicking: The Meanings of Performing and Listening.* Hanover, NH: Wesleyan University Press.

St Christopher's (2012) 'Schools Project.' Available at www.stchristophers.org.uk/public-education/schools-project, accessed on 11 June 2013.

Chapter 8

Bereavement and Loss

Gini Lawson and Nigel Hartley

Introduction

When working in a hospice or similar end of life care institution, it is inevitable that we come across people who are bereaved. There has also been much written regarding the persistent loss that those people working in the field encounter on a day to day basis and the need for planned, on-going staff support (Renzenbrink 2011).

Supporting people to draw on their own resilience and personal coping mechanisms during difficult times in their lives forms a major part of our work in end of life care. As practitioners, we also need to find useful and effective ways to both professionally and personally deal with the impact of consistently supporting and guiding people through the dying process, bereavement and loss for ourselves. Although much work has been done on developing an understanding of the theory of resilience and coping in palliative care (Monroe and Oliviere 2007), we do not fully understand why some individuals cope with adverse situations more fruitfully and successfully than others. Being able to offer a range of possibilities in order to support people through such demanding experiences is therefore essential when dealing with the unique and individual responses to death, bereavement and loss which we encounter and experience during our everyday work. Without the creative arts we lack one of the most useful mediums with which to address, contain, mould and reform people's distinct experiences of, and responses to, difficult situations such as bereavement and loss.

In this chapter, we are introduced to Gini who currently works as a community artist and as an arts therapist. Following a personal introduction, Gini focusses on the following areas:

- Working at St Christopher's

- The common stages of bereavement and loss

- How the arts can support people through bereavement and loss

- The quilting group at St Christopher's

- Healthy responses to death and dying

- A review of support structures and their importance.

The chapter concludes with some of my reflections and considerations.

Gini: my background

My name is Gini Lawson and I am often asked why I work in hospices. The truth is that I am not entirely sure how to answer the question. I have, of course, chosen to do this work, and I know that my early life has in some way prepared me for it. I know that I live differently as a consequence of the work that I do, possibly with more intensity, depth and awareness. In many ways, I have discovered my own humanity through working in hospices and I enjoy dedicating my time and energy to being with people who are dying, and to working alongside their families. I like the fact that things appear to be more real when working with people at this stage of life, and I like the intimacy of the connections that we create together. I continue to learn a lot about life and death from the people I encounter during my work.

In reality, some people assume that it is depressing to work in hospices, and some assume that I am some kind of saint or an angel. Some change the subject quickly when I begin to talk about it, and occasionally, some are intrigued to know more.

On a day to day basis, I find that death is emotionally and intellectually challenging. I have a curiosity about death and what it means to be dying and, as my work and experience become more established, I find that I am developing an inner resilience which helps me to be alongside the pain and suffering of other people. I have learned that it is important to respect the worth and individuality of each person I work with, and to assist them through an exploration of meaning, purpose and value in their life, and to sometimes create a lasting legacy through using the creative arts. One of the most important things that I have discovered is that death and loss are a very normal part of real life.

Throughout my life many of my family members have died, and I have been able to process loss and grief using the arts as a way to articulate my experiences. In 2005, I experienced a more complicated grief response. I had a molar pregnancy (a complete hydatidiform mole), which fortunately was benign. It was a difficult loss for me because I was grieving for a baby that had never actually existed, compounded by months of tests and living with the fear of cancer. I felt isolated because I had no one to speak to who had been through a similar experience. Consequently, I trained to become the first telephone support worker in the UK for people who had suffered a molar pregnancy. I was a wounded healer, and through helping others it was obvious to me that I was helping myself. Later that year I began training in integrative arts psychotherapy, and graduated with a Master's degree five years later. I am currently a registered art therapist with the Health and Care Professions Council (HCPC).

In 2006 I came across a job advertisement to work at St Christopher's Hospice as a community artist. I specifically wanted to work with people who were dying and their families because I had been so impressed by my experience of a hospice that had cared for my grandfather some years earlier. Palliative care was one of the specialisms in health care that I had not worked in, and I was attracted to the prospect of using the arts with people who were facing death. I had discovered through my own experiences of loss and bereavement that the arts can help to heal and make things better. I knew that palliative care was not curative, but could support a person to live their life to the full to the very end. I also believed that the arts could help people to achieve this.

I was successful in being offered the job at St Christopher's Hospice, and worked there throughout the period of my training as an integrative arts psychotherapist. In 2010 I qualified as an arts therapist, and, drawing on this training and my experience as a community artist, I began working in another hospice as well.

Working at St Christopher's

At St Christopher's. I work with people who are dying or who have life limiting illnesses (including cancer, a range of neurological conditions, dementia, end stage heart disease, HIV/AIDS, etc.). As with all of my colleagues at the hospice, I also work with families and carers as they live alongside their dying relative, and also work with many family members or carers after their relative has died. I facilitate open groups for patients and carers as part of the day and outpatient service, work at the bedside on the inpatient unit and in the community within people's homes and care homes. I also provide arts sessions to families when appropriate. I facilitate a weekly quilting group that is part of the St Christopher's social programme. This programme opens up the hospice to the local community in order to change attitudes both to the work of the hospice and also to what it means to be living with dying. The quilting group has an open membership which includes patients, carers, bereaved people, staff, volunteers and members of the local community. This group often sees people through the transition of being a carer to becoming a bereaved person, and then, often, beyond bereavement. I also facilitate inter-generational groups as part of our death education programme in order to promote healthier attitudes towards death and dying. The St Christopher's Schools Project, which we established in 2004, has been widely acclaimed as a useful tool to dispel myths around death and dying and rolled out both nationally and internationally. I have also worked as part of a new initiative at St Christopher's to roll out this project into local care homes.

Within the organisation, we have a strong multi-disciplinary team that is flexible and responsive to the needs of the users of our services. The team (which includes health care professionals and trained volunteers) works hard to provide a high quality service which fosters an atmosphere of generosity and respect.

The team of artists of which I am part comprises different kinds of paid arts professionals and arts students in training. We each draw on different theories to inform our approaches, and have very unique qualities.

Being an integrative arts psychotherapist I use all of the arts, namely visual arts, music, drama, movement, creative writing and sand-play therapy, and an integration of different, but complementary theories such as person-centred, existential-humanistic, psychodynamic, cognitive and behavioural. Much of the work that all of the artists are involved in focuses on meaning-making and creating lasting legacies.

Working with those who are dying brings us into close contact with families, carers and friends who inevitably also need support through loss and bereavement. As a result of working in the hospice, I, like my colleagues, experience loss and bereavement regularly, and

I am confronted with my own mortality on a daily basis. Experience has taught me that I need to support myself, seek support from my colleagues, and receive support through supervision.

I have also learned that the arts and arts therapies can provide us with useful resources throughout the bereavement process, whether for the patients themselves or for the family member or for the caregiver.

The common stages of bereavement and loss

Bereavement is an individual and universal experience that is difficult to define because of the unfathomable depth of feeling that forms loss. It is something that we experience all through life, and we sometimes need the support of others to be able to cope and move on with our lives. The various models of bereavement and loss all address the following:

- the realities of adjusting to a changed life

- the search for meaning

- the concept of a healing trajectory.

The following briefly introduces five theoretical models, which I have found useful to inform my work with bereaved people:

1. Dr Elizabeth Kubler-Ross (1970) developed the 'stages of grief' in her landmark book *On Death and Dying*. Her 'grief cycle model' describes loss from the perspective of the dying and was initially developed as a model for helping patients to cope with death and bereavement. She describes a sequential phase model of:

   - denial and isolation

   - anger

   - bargaining

   - depression

   - acceptance.

   Shock precedes stage one (*denial and isolation*) and *hope* is present from stage two (*anger*) throughout the process. Rather than a progression through the stages, she talks of a transition between them as more of an ebb and flow. The model acknowledges an individual pattern of emotional responses which people feel when coming to terms with death, loss or trauma. The model provides insight and guidance for coming to terms with personal loss and change, and for helping others with adjustment and developing coping skills. Kubler-Ross also explores the child's response to loss, and the child within the adult, to explain the unconscious processes that can be acted out.

2. The *Phase Model* (Bowlby 1980; Parkes 1986) incorporates four phases:

- shock

- yearning and protest

- despair

- recovery.

It links to attachment theory (Bowlby 1969, 1973, 1980 and 1988). Working through grief is fundamental in this model, which is understood to take place through the four overlapping phases. Working through these phases is understood to enable detachment (the breaking of the affectional bonds) and reorganisation (the continuation of the bond with the deceased). An altered attachment to the deceased allows for a gradual adjustment to the physical absence of the deceased person in the bereaved person's on-going life.

3. The *Task Model* (Worden 1991) is widely used in the planning of therapeutic interventions for bereaved people. It describes four tasks required for an adjustment to bereavement:

- accepting the reality of loss

- experiencing the pain of grief

- adjusting to an environment without the deceased

- relocating the deceased and moving on with life.

It presents a dynamic process whereby the bereaved person actively struggles to work through grief, rather than passively experiencing it. The model suggests that a bereaved person may not necessarily work through all the tasks or in any sequential order.

4. The *Dual Process Model of Coping with Bereavement* (Stroebe and Schut 1999) builds upon and extends both the phase model and task model. It is a model of a nuanced approach to adaptive coping. It takes into consideration the following:

- complicated grief

- gender differences

- the social and cultural context of grieving

- the time dimension.

The model describes two categories of stressors associated with bereavement, and a process of oscillation between them that is characteristic of 'normal' bereavement. The categories are:

- loss-orientation

- restoration-orientation.

The principle underlying the process of oscillation is that at times the bereaved person will confront aspects of loss, while at other times will avoid them, implying that coping with bereavement is a complex regulatory process of confrontation and avoidance. The model proposes that the oscillation process is necessary for the achievement of adaptive coping. Like the phase model, it also has a strong link with attachment theory, and predicts that people with different attachment styles will cope with grief differently; people with a *secure* attachment style are more likely to oscillate more easily between loss- and restoration-orientations; people with an *ambivalent* attachment style might be more exclusively loss-orientated and may experience chronic grieving; people with an *avoidant* attachment style are likely to be more restoration-orientated, delaying or inhibiting their grief; and people with an *insecure* attachment style may have a more disturbed and less coherent manner of oscillating between loss- and restoration-orientations (Stroebe 2008).

5. More recently, two psychologists Okun and Nowinski (2011) make the case that advances in diagnosis and treatment enabling people to live longer with life-threatening illnesses have significantly changed the bereavement process. Their book *Saying Goodbye: How Families Can Find Renewal Through Loss* suggests that prolonged crisis changes the pattern of grief encountered by families who face the loss of a loved one through protracted illness. Drawing on the authors' personal experiences of loss and other's experiences of loss, they propose that the following stages begin long before a person actually dies:

- crisis and anxiety

- unity

- upheaval

- resolution

- renewal.

The book argues that the way we grieve has changed since 1970 because death now refers to a process rather than an event because people are dying differently. It acknowledges the peaks and troughs of hope and despair along the trajectory of a terminal illness as a person may go in and out of remission, or undergo different treatment trials. If the affectional bond is not strong, feelings can expand to include guilt or anger in the *crisis and anxiety* stage; fractious relationships require a setting aside of past differences and pulling together in the *unity* stage; throughout the *upheaval* stage unity can wear thin as caregivers can experience burnout; the *resolution* stage provides opportunities to confront long-standing issues and redefinition of one's role in the family; the final stage, *renewal*, begins with the funeral and continues as individuals adjust to loss and bereavement, and to their changed roles.

While these theories are very helpful for both legitimising feelings and developing approaches to working through grief, my experience shows me that death and loss are a singularly personal experience coloured by individual life experience, beliefs and culture, relationships and time.

How the arts can support people through bereavement and loss

The idea that the arts can be helpful in processing loss and enabling and supporting mourning is certainly not new. The desire to use the arts during grief has been explored by many (Dissanayake 1988; Hatcher 1985; Peckman 1965). Whatever the theoretical explanation, it is clear that the arts somehow help us to cope with the trauma of death. The arts can provide a context to contain and potentially alleviate feelings of anxiety, fear, crisis and threat (Johnson 1987). They can be used to mark the significance of death through the creation of visual and musical rituals (Dissanayake 1988). The arts are known to have been used in funeral ceremonies since Neanderthal times. Funerals, as a universal human experience, incorporate symbolic solutions to contain emotions, and aesthetic solutions to release emotions (Hatcher 1985). It is probable that we have never been to, and may never go to, a funeral without music, poetry or flowers.

We are told that in years gone by, communities came together to support those who experienced a death in the family (Rosenblatt, Walsh and Jackson 1976). Today, individuals are often isolated from extended family members and the community (Platt and Persico 1992), resulting in bereaved people feeling alone and lacking basic and adequate support (Rodgers and Cowles 1991).

The creative arts feature heavily as part of the St Christopher's social programme and aim to offer individuals the opportunity to share thoughts, feelings and experiences with others.

I have learned that death is a social experience, and that a person's death is influenced by the communities within which they live. With the arts at the heart of the St Christopher's social programme, an effective outlet for loss is made possible through a shared community experience. This promotes healthier attitudes towards death and dying, loss and change, because it locates death and loss back into the community where it belongs. Hospices have a responsibility to educate society (DH 2008), and using the arts and working with myths and metaphors enables a context not only to express feelings and gain support, but also a context which offers a social learning experience.

Benefits from group involvement include increased emotional, and also mental and physical stability during and after participation (McCallum, Piper and Morin 1993; Yalom and Vinogradov 1988). More specific benefits of group participation include:

- expressing emotions and developing better stress management skills

- coping with loneliness and developing support systems

- improving self-esteem.

The benefits of group work can be increased with the use of the arts (Raymer and McIntyre 1987; Schimmel and Kornreich 1993) and are well-suited to the needs of bereaved people (Aldridge 1993; Malchiodi 1991). This is because many individuals are unable to fully express their sense of grief through words as often there is not a common language to talk about such difficult issues. The arts, therefore, offer a unique context for non-verbal expression (Borden 1992; Simon 1981; Zambelli and DeRosa 1992). Through engagement with the arts in a group context, individuals can express themselves in new ways and discover new resources to cope with loss and change (Grant 1995; Graves 1994).

My experience shows me that art-making promotes a sense of joy, peace and relaxation, as well as offering a place to struggle with focus and determination. This experience in a social context creates a powerful group resonance and a place for positive, energising and meaningful encounters. With a dual emphasis on process and product creation, participants are rewarded for their efforts with a final product which provides insight into, and a record of, the process, as well as a lasting legacy (Schimmel and Kornreich 1993). When a person is attempting to assimilate loss, the permanence of an art object (whether this is a poem, image, film, music recording, story or quilt) may provide comfort (Irwin 1991). Baker (1991) states that the arts provide a concrete memorial which gives the author or artist a unique place in the world. The finished product may be witnessed over time, which allows for a continued resonance and lasting legacy.

It is thought that many bereaved people are able to express themselves more readily using creative arts therapies than through traditional talking therapies (Irwin 1991; Junge 1985; McIntyre 1990; Simon 1981). Given that many of us find it difficult to find the words to articulate thoughts and emotions associated with loss and grief, we may need to utilise something new and different in order to articulate ourselves (Simon 1981). People may also struggle to know what to say to someone who is bereaved. The arts seem to be a natural ally when words are difficult to find (Raymer and McIntyre 1987).

Many arts therapists and artists have described and researched the use of creative expression with those who have experienced loss (Junge 1985; Raymer and McIntyre 1987; Simon 1981; Speert 1992). Arts therapists and artists consistently observe the power and potential of the arts to identify, cope with, and heal the pain experienced in grief (Forrest and Thomas 1991; Grant 1995; Graves 1994; Orton 1994). The number of articles about arts therapies with the dying and bereaved has steadily risen in hospice and arts therapies literature over the past 20 years or so, evidencing the value of non-verbal creative therapeutic approaches (Bertman 1999; Birnbaum 1991; Crenshaw 1990; Goldstein, Alter and Axelrod 1996; Levi, Gilad and Friedman-Kalmovitca 1996).

The St Christopher's quilting project

The St Christopher's quilting project provides people with a creative outlet, and the group setting provides individuals with the opportunity to connect with others in a relatively informal atmosphere, thereby reducing social isolation and the withdrawal from society of those that are reluctant (for whatever reason) to engage in more formal bereavement groups. The context of the group promotes healthier attitudes towards death and dying as participants also have the opportunity to become comfortable alongside others at all stages and phases of life and death. The sharing of creative work augments and deepens the connections between individuals, particularly if a group quilt is being created, as each person's piece is joined together, becoming an integrated whole. These important interactions between group participants, myself as the facilitator, and the process of quilting supports all of us to move from isolation and loneliness to connection and empowerment, from denial to acceptance, from loss of control and anxiety to relief, from disintegration to integration, and from despair to hope. Quilt making, as with all of the arts, by nature of its two-phase process of expression and reflection, allows for both the intimacy of internal focus and the external communication and connection with others. As symbols of loss and change are shared with others in the group, a deeper understanding of oneself and the development of empathy with others can evolve. Participants have the opportunity to demonstrate these elements of co-operation, creativity and re-creating of their internal world through external experimentation. The group also provides reflective possibilities to both contain and mirror each individual's experience of loss and validate his or her sense of self (Birnbaum 1991).

As part of the quilting group, quilts are often made in memory of someone who has died as a means to remember or commemorate what has been lost (Graves 1994). Numerous participants have made quilts from the deceased person's clothing. The group, being open and inclusive, can also support people through anticipatory grief. Several participants have joined the group as carers because of wanting to have a support group in place after their loved one dies. Some participants use the arts to promote a sense of unity and legacy. A young mother and her daughter made a quilt together, so that when the mother died, the daughter had something to connect her to her mother.

When I recently conducted an evaluation, participants placed a high value on the relationships within the group. The atmosphere of the hospice was also valued, as it was experienced as a welcoming place, and a number of people commented on the experience of feeling accepted. The process of quilting was also recognised to be an important therapeutic factor, being described as relaxing, releasing, relieving, and rewarding.

> I feel like you helped me so much when you reached out to me after my husband's death and helped me channel all my energy and sadness into art. Thank you. (a quote from the quilting group evaluation)

Without proper support for both the expression and containment of feelings related to loss, people can suffer with low self-esteem, depression, suicidal ideation and physical illness (Stroebe and Stroebe 1987; Vachon *et al.* 1982). Some people who are bereaved will need supportive interventions in order to prevent long-term health problems. For many, short-term support can be useful in order to help people re-engage with life. The social programme is a very low cost, yet effective supportive intervention. Participants are free to decide to what level they wish to engage with this service, without expectations from the organisation. Additionally there are more short-term, intensive and formal bereavement interventions available for those who need to access these.

Case study: supporting individuals through loss and bereavement

Perhaps one of my most memorable experiences of working with a bereaved person was with Sam. Sam was in her early thirties and her boyfriend had died of cancer. Sam was referred for art therapy and used the sessions to tell her story through images and art objects, while reminiscing over her life with her boyfriend, and his death. She recalled the story of when they first met, and many other stories of their lives together, some amusing and some sad. I would describe her images as both embodied and symbolic, such as a withering plant wrenched out of soil and a candle without a flame. Some were depictions of her struggling to stay afloat in a vast sea, her falling into a black hole, her weeping over his grave, her in an empty bed. In one session she painted a picture of her garden, full of flowers. When she gave voice to the image, she said that the garden was missing her boyfriend and the children that they had hoped to have. She was very tearful as she described her grief for the children they would never have. She chose to take this image home with her as she wanted to show it to her mum. She came back the following week and said that the image had been very useful as it had helped her to talk about one of the most painful parts of her grief with her mum. She said that the image had allowed her to start the conversations that she needed to have in order to let out the pain. She worked on a new image of the garden, this time with children in it. She said that, although she could not imagine falling in love with someone new, she could imagine that one day she may have children.

According to Simon (1981), art created during bereavement can represent an attempt to work through conflicts and usually occurs in three overlapping stages:

- expression of the conflict

- arts as container

- resolution.

My work with Sam reminds me of this process. The first stage brings closer to consciousness the feelings that lie behind the sense of dis-ease. In the second stage the arts provide an image/metaphor that enables the suffering of the first stage to find containment as it is gradually transformed into mourning. The third stage brings resolution as one comes to view death as a natural end, and therefore one is better resourced for coping with life.

In summary, the creative experience of making art during a time of loss provides an opportunity for self-exploration and transformation. Art-making allows the bereaved person to focus inward and express emotions in a way that feels manageable. This can help prevent some of the psychological, social and behavioural problems resulting from unresolved grief. In addition, the value of undertaking bereavement support as part of a compassionate community where people are welcoming and supportive can only be enhanced by the process of creativity.

Healthy responses to death and dying

We know instinctively that it is healthy to acknowledge death and dying, loss and change as part of life, and the best death educators in our society must surely be the people who are actually dying. It is therefore important to support people and to provide opportunities for those people using our services to promote healthier attitudes towards hospices, death and dying outwards into the communities within which we live. The St Christopher's Schools Project brings children and young people together with people who are dying and, through engaging together through the arts, we learn a great deal from both patients, family members and the children and young people who take part. Children often ask direct questions and can elicit straightforward and uncomplicated answers. Children have asked questions such as 'what is it like to have no hair?' and 'what is it like to be dying?' Our evaluation processes tell us that patients have found these questions refreshing, because they are not the sort of questions that adults usually dare to ask, yet they are real questions that relate to dying and loss and need to be expressed. The openness of the children facilitates openness from patients, which can bring about a huge sense of respite and release.

Death is neither played down nor played up during these schools projects. It is not romanticised, nor is it denied. The hospice is not portrayed as a house of death, and feedback from participants tells us that they see more life in the building than anywhere else. I think that there is sometimes criticism towards hospices for appearing to be lively places and that they are sometimes misunderstood because they seem joyous. The problem is that this liveliness can be misinterpreted as a façade, and a denial of death. The reality, from my own experience, is that life and death are one continuum and both contain unfathomable depths of feeling. Life and death, when experienced to the full, contain an appreciation of, and a commitment to, what matters most. There is no life without death and there is no death without life. If hospices are a true reflection of community, then both will be present in equal measure.

We often receive feedback from our users and visitors to the hospice, stating their surprise to find that their expectations of the hospice are in stark contrast to their experience in reality. People expect an atmosphere of distress and depression, and instead experience something very different. I myself sometimes experience a sense of gratitude for life which sits alongside the distress and despair of death and loss. However, for some people, denying the fact that they are dying may be the only way that they can carry on living. There is no doubt for me, that for these people, this is a healthy response to their situation, and I have learned that we need to let people live their dying in their own way.

A review of support structures and their importance

Most health care organisations will have both formal and informal mechanisms for support. There may be group supervision on offer as there is at St Christopher's, where all members of the multi-disciplinary team have the opportunity to meet together with a skilled external supervisor. There should also be managerial supervision with a line manager and regular multi-disciplinary team meetings, as well as more informal collegial support. As individuals, we are all responsible for self-care and looking after ourselves, and we will all discover our own ways of doing this. As a creative person first and foremost, I have found that it is important not to overlook my own art-making, as this is the most important resource available to me for processing feelings associated with loss and bereavement. As well as the emotional and psychological benefits, it also keeps creativity alive within myself and my own relationship with creativity is important to keep investing in, both for my own support and development and for that of the people with whom I work.

As an arts therapist you will be registered with the Health and Care Professions Council, and you will have a professional responsibility to engage in regular clinical supervision. If you are training to be an arts therapist, you will be required to have regular supervision for your work at your placements. If you are an artist (community or arts in health practitioner) you will also need to take such things seriously. When working with loss and bereavement, I think it is an imperative that we seek formal sources of support. The impact of loss can at times be huge, because we form deep attachments to people who die, no matter how experienced at maintaining a professional distance we may be.

I can recall a time when I was grief stricken by the death of a patient and her grieving husband. I was mourning for a young couple who were so much in love. Many emotions flooded me and I feared that I could drown in the tears that came from deep inside me. I was weeping in my supervision session, and I felt a combination of relief and shame. I felt the shame of what I assumed must have been burnout. My supervisor sat calmly with me, and mentioned that this was something that we all go through at times, and that it was quite normal. I would occasionally weep at my desk for some days later, and my colleagues would be around and they would support me when necessary. I felt a terrible sense of guilt because the young woman had died quite suddenly, and no one was quite expecting it. I had been planning with her an exhibition of the artwork we had created together and I berated myself for not timing this better, as if I should have known that she was going to die when she did. I shared this with her husband, which enabled him to share his own sense of guilt. He then asked that we go ahead with the exhibition in honour of his wife. The opening night was attended by friends and family, doctors, nurses and other staff as well as volunteers and fundraisers. There was no doubt that this was a cathartic process for all of us present, including myself, as we reflected on what this young woman had meant to each of us.

However 'professional' we are in our work, my experience has shown me that the emotional surges we encounter on a daily basis can sometimes take their toll and it is important to acknowledge them as part of a normal process and seek support when needed. These experiences have also helped me to become more resilient and robust.

My intention has been to give an overview of some theory and some personal examples from practice. Loss and bereavement are an inevitable and challenging part of life. For me, these experiences are also enriching, developing a fuller appreciation of life and love, a deepening of relationships to myself and others, a development of resilience and robustness. Perhaps the most striking observation from my own practice is that the arts help to gain a perspective that has the right balance of emotional distance and emotional connection to allow for movement through and beyond grief. The process requires full presence in the moment, allowing for some relief from rumination and associated feelings of anger and guilt that are so commonplace with loss. These, sometimes overwhelming, feelings can become manageable as they emerge and are transformed through a process utilising the creative arts where a retrieval and renewal of life can be activated.

Reflection

Each one of us will die, and we will all be bereaved (Monroe and Oliviere 2007). During our lives, we will experience the challenges and struggles of coming to terms with loss, whether through the death of someone we love, or through losing something in a more general sense. Experiencing loss or bereavement can challenge the very essence of who we are and what we believe to be important in life. Supporting someone through the dying process can also lead us to ask the big questions such as what is life all about and why do we, and the people we care for, need to suffer? As Gini mentions, these things can, and will, sometimes take their toll. Yet, for the majority of us, through accessing some basic, time-limited support, we can straightforwardly discover previously unidentified ways of coping, which can not only help us through the traumatic times, but can enable us to imagine and experience ourselves anew as part of an altered future.

Each one of us will bring our own experiences of bereavement and loss to working in end of life care, as well as our own fears about death and dying, some of which might be buried deep within our unconscious. What we hear from Gini, and what I have learned from my own experience is that developing an acute sense of self-awareness is a necessity when working in end of life care. There is no use pretending to ourselves and others that all is well, when in reality we are feeling vulnerable, alone and afraid. Although it is common, and sometimes trite, to translate the intense feelings which we carry with us from our work into psychological theory and firmly place the blame for our state of mind at the door of those people we care for and work with, in reality, much of the emotional confusion that we experience comes from deep within ourselves.

When I began working at London Lighthouse, the UK's first centre for people living with HIV/AIDS over 20 years ago, I found myself arriving at work early and walking up and down the street before being able to pluck up the courage to enter the building. This experience filled me with both puzzlement and anxiety. Why was it so difficult to walk through a door into my place of work? Was I simply doing the wrong job? It did not take long to realise that my own fears, experiences and expectations were getting in the way of what was, in reality, a job of work. I had recently looked after a friend who had died of an AIDS-related illness and I was also terrified of the possibility of confronting my own death. To be of help to people who were dying, to people who were afraid and vulnerable, I had to learn to be able to get myself out of the way; after all it was not my dying, it was theirs, and through my work I was committing myself to supporting them and to be of use to them during their dying process. You will have seen that this process of getting ourselves out of the way is discussed in more detail in Chapter 2.

Experiencing my own bereavement and being afraid of dying myself was not wrong, but when working with people who are dying or bereaved such things need to be acknowledged, understood and managed. I believe that we are consistently confronting ourselves within the work that we do with those people who are dying or who are bereaved on a daily basis, and we need to discover ways of being generous enough to let the people we care for claim their own dying process, not getting in their way and gently supporting them when needed; a tremendously demanding and complex task.

Getting ourselves out of the way is not an easy process, and for some people I have seen that it is just not possible. This usually manifests itself in hospice workers as a consistent need for personal self-support, where nothing ever seems to be enough. As we see from Gini's account, for many people bereavement and loss is, and should be, regarded as a normal process. When we experience loss and bereavement, for the greater part of us our responses and reactions to these life-changing events will be expected, healthy and manageable. With a limited, concentrated and cost effective package of support, the majority of us will be able to move on with our lives with the confidence and competence we need, and we see that the creative arts can be a useful way of achieving this. Only a minority of people will require support which is more on-going, controlled and in-depth (Hartley 2008).

As people who work with the dying, regular, planned supervision should be ample and adequate and if we find that we cannot move on from our experiences in order to continue to be helpful to the next group of people who need our support, we are probably in trouble. There is a danger in thinking that working with people who are dying or who are bereaved is the most difficult job in the world. In reality, it is no more easy nor more difficult than the next job and neither should it be.

People ask how we can cope with working in hospices. This is possibly because they are personally afraid of death, have been bereaved themselves or are just curious and are, in some way, processing their own experiences. We should not seek support just for support's sake; what I mean by this is just because we are told that working with dying and bereaved people should be difficult, we must not fall into the trap of satisfying other people's curiosity. How do I cope with working in a hospice? Far more than any formal process of support and supervision, the reality is that I have consistently been refreshed by going out for a good meal with my family, by meeting friends in the pub, by cycling and going to the gym and by grabbing a bargain in the New Year sales. On the rare occasion when something more is needed, I seek out a colleague.

References

Aldridge, D. (1993) 'Hope, meaning and the creative arts therapies in the treatment of grief.' *The Arts in Psychotherapy 20*, 285–297.

Baker, S.R. (1991) 'Utilizing Art and Imagery in Death and Dying Counselling.' In D. Papadatou and C. Papadatos (eds) *Children and Death: Series in Death Education, Aging & Health*. New York, NY: Hemisphere Publishing.

Bertman, S. (1999) *Grief and the Healing Arts: Creativity as Therapy*. New York: Baywood Publishing Company Inc.

Birnbaum, B. (1991) 'Haven hugs and bugs: An innovative multiple-family weekend intervention for bereaved children adolescents and adults.' *American Journal of Hospice and Palliative Care 8*, 5, 23–9.

Borden, G. (1992) 'Metaphor: Visual aid in grief work.' *Omega 25*, 3, 239–248.

Bowlby, J. (1969) *Attachment and Loss. Vol 1, Attachment*. Harmondsworth: Penguin.

Bowlby, J. (1973) *Attachment and Loss. Vol 2, Separation; Anxiety and Anger*. Harmondsworth: Penguin.

Bowlby, J. (1980) *Attachment and Loss. Vol 3, Loss; Sadness and Depression*. Harmondsworth: Penguin.

Bowlby, J. (1988) *A Secure Base: Clinical Applications of Attachment Theory*. Didcot: Routledge.

Crenshaw, D.A. (1990) *Bereavement: Counselling the Grieving Throughout the Life Cycle*. New York: Continuum Publishing.

DH (Department of Health) (2008). *End of Life Care Strategy: Promoting High Quality Care for All Adults at the End of Life*. London: DH.

Dissanayake, E. (1988) *What is Art For?* Seattle, WA: University of Washington Press.

Forrest, M. and Thomas G.V. (1991) 'An exploratory study of drawings by bereaved children.' *British Journal of Clinical Psychology 30*, 4, 373–4.

Goldstein, J., Alter, C.L. and Axelrod, R.A. (1996) 'Psychoeducational bereavement support group for families provided in an out-patient cancer centre.' *Journal of Cancer Education 11*, 4, 233–237.

Grant, A. (1995) *The Healing Journey: Manual for a Grief Support Group*. Long Branch, NJ: Vista Publishing.

Graves, S. (1994) *Expressions of Healing*. Van Nuys, CA: New Castle Publishing.

Hartley, N. (2008) 'The arts in health and social care – is music therapy fit for purpose?' *British Journal of Music Therapy 22*, 2, 88–96.

Hatcher, E. (1985) *Art as Culture*. Landham, MD: University Press of America.

Irwin, H.J. (1991) 'The depiction of loss: Use of clients' drawings in bereavement counselling.' *Death Studies 15*, 481–497.

Johnson, D.R. (1987) 'The role of the creative arts therapies in the diagnosis and treatment of trauma.' *The Arts in Psychotherapy 14*, 7–13.

Junge, M. (1985) 'The book about Daddy dying: A preventive art therapy technique to help families deal with the death of a family member.' *Art Therapy: Journal of the American Art Therapy Association 2*, 1, 410–419.

Kubler-Ross, E. (1970) *On Death and Dying*. London: Tavistock.

Levi, S., Gilad, R. and Friedman-Kalmovitca, A. (1996) 'Pictorial art as a teaching strategy in death education.' *Nursing Times Research 1*, 3, 198–205.

Malchiodi, C.A. (1991) 'Art and loss.' *Art Therapy: Journal of the American Art Therapy Association 9*, 3, 114–118.

McCallum, M., Piper, W. E. and Morin, H. (1993) 'Affect and outcome in short term group therapy for loss.' *Nursing Research 47*, 2–10.

McIntyre, B.B. (1990) 'Art Therapy with bereaved youth.' *Journal of Palliative Care, 6*, 1, 16–25.

Monroe, B. and Oliviere, D. (2007) *Resilience in Palliative Care – Achievement in Adversity*. Oxford: Oxford University Press.

Okun, B. and Nowinski, J. (2011) *Saying Goodbye: How Families Can Find Renewal Through Loss*. Boston, MA: Harvard Health Publications.

Orton, M. (1994) 'A case study of an adolescent mother grieving the death of her child due to Sudden Infant Death Syndrome.' *Art Therapy: American Journal of Art Therapy 33*, 2, 37–44.

Parkes, C.M. (1986) *Bereavement: Studies of Grief in Adult Life*. New York: Basic Books.

Peckman, M. (1965) *Man's Rage for Chaos: Biology, Behavior and the Arts*. Philadelphia, PA: Chilton.

Platt, L. and Persico, V.R. (1992) *Grief in Cross-cultural Perspective: A Casebook*. New York: Garland Publishing.

Raymer, M. and McIntyre, B.B. (1987) 'An art support group for bereaved children and adolescents.' *Art Therapy Journal of the American Art Therapy Association 4*, 27–35.

Renzenbrink, I. (2011) *Caregiver Stress and Staff Support in Illness, Dying and Bereavement*. Oxford: Oxford University Press.

Rodgers, B.L. and Cowles, K.V. (1991) 'The concept of grief: An analysis of classical and contemporary thought.' *Death Studies 15*, 5, 443–459.

Rosenblatt, P.C., Walsh, R.R., and Jackson, D.A. (1976) *Grief and Mourning in Cross-cultural Perspective*. New Haven, CT: Human Relations Area Files.

Schimmel, B.F. and Kornreich, T.Z. (1993) 'The use of art and verbal process with recently widowed individuals.' *American Journal of Art Therapy 31*, 91–97.

Simon, R. (1981) 'Bereavement art.' *American Journal of Art Therapy 20*, 135–143.

Speert, E. (1992) 'The use of art therapy following perinatal death.' *Art Therapy: Journal of the American Art Therapy Association 9*, 3, 121–128.

Stroebe, M. (2008) 'The dual process model of coping with bereavement: Overview and Update.' *Grief Matters 11*, 1, 4–10.

Stroebe, M.S. and Schut, H. (1999) 'The dual process model of coping with bereavement: rationale and description.' *Death Studies 23*, 3, 197–224.

Stroebe, W. and Stroebe, M.S. (1987) *Bereavement and Health*. New York: Cambridge University Press.

Vachon, M.L.S., Sheldon, A.R., Lancee, W.J., Lyall, W.A.L., Rogers, J., and Freeman, S.J.J. (1982) 'Correlates of enduring distress patterns following bereavement: Social network, life situation, and personality.' *Psychological Medicine 12*, 783–788.

Worden, J.W. (1991) *Grief Counselling and Grief Therapy: A Handbook for the Mental Health Practitioner.* 2nd Edition. New York: Springer Publishing Company.

Yalom, I. and Vinogradov, S. (1988) 'Bereavement groups: Techniques and themes.' *International Journal of Group Psychotherapy 38*, 4, 419–457.

Zambelli, G.C. and DeRosa, A.P. (1992) 'Bereavement support groups for school age children: Theory, intervention and case example.' *American Journal of Orthopsychiatry 62*, 4, 484–93.

PART 3

Starting Out, Looking After Yourself, Research and Development

Chapter 9

Getting Started

Roberto Marcelo Sánchez-Camus and Nigel Hartley

Introduction

Making a decision to put oneself forward for a new job, filling out an application form and attending an interview can be somewhat of a daunting prospect.

- What is it that attracts us to a certain position?

- Is it an area that we have worked in before?

- Do we want a new experience in a different area of health care? Will this be our first job after training?

- Is it just because new jobs are scarce and we are applying for everything that comes along?

The answers to all of the above questions will challenge and motivate each of us in different ways and will impact on how we put ourselves across to a prospective employer, both in writing as part of an application form and also in person should we be called for interview.

Starting out in a new position also raises a number of other questions which can challenge us both personally and professionally. These questions will include:

- Do I believe in the ethos of the organisation?

- Who will be my manager?

- Will my expectations be the same as my employer's?

- What will the organisation's relationship with the arts and therapies be like?

- Will people like me, and will I do well?

- What will be the barriers to prevent things working well?

During the main part of this chapter we hear from Roberto, who is an experienced community artist. Following some information about his background, Roberto focusses on the following:

- Interviews, presentations and what to expect

- Beginning a new job and project planning

- An example of a project outline

- Implementing a project: making it work

- Working within the frameworks of institutions

- Working in partnership with other institutions

- Working alongside other health care professionals

- Two important challenges

- Changing culture.

Roberto shares some short stories with us to illustrate some of the key points raised. The chapter concludes with my reflections and considerations.

Roberto: my background

My name is Roberto Marcelo Sánchez-Camus and I have discovered that working in end of life care can be a unique and extraordinary experience for a creative arts practitioner. As an artist, I have worked in a variety of educational settings both in community and academic contexts. While completing my PhD in Applied Live Art, I sought part-time employment as an arts facilitator doing socially engaged work. Always interested in the interstices between creativity and community, I found my interests in art-making and social activism worked best when combined in a community setting where I could bring the arts to those who may not necessarily have access to them. St Christopher's was seeking a community artist to join their existing team of artists. The call sought among other things 'an exceptional individual to develop and maintain a flexible community arts service for patients and carers...as well as developing a series of art exhibitions and partnerships with other arts organisations...' The position required a practising artist who had his or her own portfolio as well as experience of working in a community context. Though I had never worked in end of life care I had developed and implemented community projects with young people and adults in a variety of social settings. I knew that I had the artistic skills combined with the teaching experience to run workshops and to create exhibitions. Furthermore like many artists working in today's media saturated environment, I had multiple skills that included traditional painting, drawing and sculpture as well as filming, editing and performance. Considering my skill range and interest in broadening the scope of my community work, I decided to apply to St Christopher's, although I had no previous experience in end of life care and had never been to a hospice before. My goal was to present my qualifications as an artist and an educator, and demonstrate my willingness to expand my knowledge of community work into end of life care.

Interviews, presentations and what to expect

St Christopher's offered me an interview and requested that I present an arts project that I had developed and led. I created a PowerPoint presentation of a project I had run in West Africa with two groups of young people, around the topic of HIV/AIDS prevention. I also used some short two-minute DVD footage of the work being created in order to showcase the project in its actuality. I chose this project because it was related to health care and it was the most recent and large-scale community project I had completed. As with any interview I prepared as much as I could, by reading about the history and services at St Christopher's, visiting the website and recapping how their job description might fit my experience and qualifications. Communication for me is easy and relaxed and I am someone comfortable with job interviews. In retrospect I realise that though I could read about the history of the hospice movement, the actual reality of working in end of life care was much different.

In reality I had very little idea what this new phase of professional development was or would mean to me both as an artist and as an individual. The interview itself was the first realisation of this. Though I felt confident to answer all the questions as honestly as possible, they were very difficult given the tender subject of death and dying. My recommendation for the reader is that prior to preparing for an interview in a hospice setting it is important to consider one's own relationship to the death process. For my own part I intellectualised the phenomena beforehand and it was only during the interview that I had to come to terms with the reality of where I was attempting to position myself. I recall one question that asked me to explain what my relationship with death was. The question seemed brutal in its context yet wholly necessary, and I found myself completely unprepared to answer.

Though it would seem obvious to have given a thought to one's own relationship to death before interviewing to work at a hospice, I have found that most people deny this relationship, even many who find themselves dying. In order to answer the question, my own thoughts recalled the recent death of a family member and my relationship to the procedures of dying. I realised that in a sense I could be quite analytical about death and dying, though that realisation came in my honest recollection of my own way of dealing with the situation. Other topics which seemed important to note are being prepared to deal with urgent situations should they arise, collaboration with a larger team of support staff, and thinking around why it is important to integrate a creative arts practice as part of a managed death process. My interview to be a community artist at St Christopher's is now archived in my memory as one of the more difficult ones I have sat through, less due to the interpersonal dynamic at the table and more due to the self-reflection I was faced with and in many ways unprepared for. I was given a tour of the hospice after the interview, my first time visiting such facilities. Following the interview, I had the distinct impression that the job was much more difficult than I could have ever imagined and that my own high energy and optimistic outlook may not have matched what they were seeking in the position. I was definitely wrong; that afternoon I was offered the position and embarked on a journey that changed my perception of death and dying and which has added a valuable asset to my skill set as an artist and a teacher.

To recap:

- Ask for an informal visit to the organisation before the interview.

- Show your work and tell stories as part of the interview – show arts objects, digital media, share case studies etc.

- Make sure that the presentation material is relevant to the setting.

- Look at the organisational website to inform your interview.

- Read about the context – death, bereavement and the creative arts.

- Include relevant information to show that you have researched the background both of the work and the organisation.

- Pre-think questions that you might be asked – particularly around your own relationship with death and how this might affect your ability both to perform at the interview and to carry out the job.

Beginning a new job and project planning

Working at St Christopher's is exceptionally rewarding and at times quite challenging. At the time of my arrival, the institution was undergoing a massive structural redevelopment, opening a new state of the art day and outpatient centre, which is now called the Anniversary Centre. This refurbishment modernised the setting of the hospice in a bold and important way. The old day centre room, where outpatients mingled, at times together with inpatients who were capable of attending, had been built in the 1980s and, though modernised, remained tethered to the aesthetic of the era. Beige and carpeted with window shades and floral patterns, it is a look that I have encountered in countless care institutions across the country. I was lucky enough to work both within that setting and also within the new centre, which opened a year after my arrival. The new centre is a spacious multi-format meeting place and café, with an espresso bar, a help desk, internet stations and a wall of full glass doors that overlook a well-designed garden. The old sense of the extended home lounge with the curtains drawn has been replaced with a light-filled modern hub, that feels energetic, open and yet comfortable. This change is important, as it is one of the aspects of St Christopher's that makes it quite unique to the other institutions I have encountered. St Christopher's also has a dedicated art pavilion surrounded by gardens and light. A large maze of interconnected buildings, and at the time I began working undergoing renovation, meant that getting my bearings was quite a challenge in the beginning. I now wish I had spent more time getting to know the building at the beginning of my work.

I was accustomed to educational and health and social care settings where most of the time was spent running a workshop, preceded by a short time for preparation and then finally completing an assessment or outcomes quickly. Working as part of a group of artists and arts therapists delivering arts projects to patients, this allocation of time changed. Outcome, assessment and referrals are an important aspect to the work, for the time spent developing the project with patients leads to many insights into their relationship to dying which can sometimes need referrals to other members of the multi-disciplinary team for more in-depth support.

To run a successful arts project it is also important to have the correct materials at hand, thus always ordering and stocking reserves of supplies in advance of the project itself. It is crucial to take into consideration the varying abilities of patients, some of whom have restricted motor skills, thus a variety of materials may be needed for the same workshop to accommodate these different needs. To begin you may create projects with the materials at hand, but the most successful works are, like any creative artworks, prepared well in advance with materials ordered and an outlined workshop plan in place. In my role as a community artist my projects took on two forms, larger-scale works with groups of patients and then smaller projects working one to one with a patient and/or carer. Generally when working one to one what was to be created as the final project was a negotiation between the person's interests and myself as the community artist and arts facilitator. This could take on the form of simple watercolours where the person may want to copy an image, or perhaps I might suggest creating an image from memory or even just to play with colour and line.

Case study: a multi-media bedtime story

With one patient I created a more complex project over a period of time where he narrated a bedtime story he would tell to his children. I recorded the story and transcribed it as well as helping him to illustrate images from key moments of the narrative. In the end we created a book with the text and images complete with an audio recording of his voice reading the book.

An example of a project outline

When running group projects I have learned that it is important to have a structure planned and written out in advance. There are many ways to create a structure and I offer as an example my own outline:

Table 9.1: Example outline of a project

Example Outline of Project Structure
Title of project:
It is always good to have a name for a workshop, especially as many of the workshops should aim to end in an exhibition or presentation of the work, thus there is already a working title. It helps contextualise the process.
Technique:
Simply the media which is being used with a description of the format. For example: acrylic painting, still life, documentary filmmaking with digital video, etc.
Purpose/concepts:
What the project is exploring. Some examples I have used are: exploring memory associations through colour and texture with watercolours, or creating puppets that represent street sellers in old London and discussing the ways the city has changed.
Project key words:
This is helpful for you as the facilitator to engage with visual/aural vocabulary, which we can sometimes take for granted as an artist but can be very new material for people who possibly have not done a hands on arts project since childhood. Examples may be simple or complex and relate to technique or concept: narrative, dreams, depth, abstraction, editing, frame, contour, etc. These key words will situate the project and help you explain the process.
Materials:
Plan out all your materials in advance. A simple watercolour painting with a group of 20 may require: 40 sheets of 11" x 18" textured watercolour paper, 3 x ½" masking tape, 10 sets of watercolour paints, 20 thick watercolour brushes, 20 thin detail brushes, 10 containers for water, 2 x buckets/1 with clean water, 1 empty to dispose dirty water, 3 x rolls paper towel, 10 plastic aprons, 4 printed examples of other works, 2 x semi-completed examples on same paper used in workshop.
Activity:
In this section you expand on the technique, now describing exactly what the project will be. For example, if we take documentary filmmaking we may put in activity: patients will work with facilitator and volunteers to come up with interview questions for each other and for staff members in the care home. They will learn the basics of using a digital video recorder and then take turns recording each other and interviewing each other, as well as staff and friends and family who may be present. The final film will be edited into a video for an invited screening celebration.

cont.

Motivation/intro:
Getting started is the hardest part. This section allows you to kick-start the workshop by delineating how you introduce what the project will be. You may show examples of other completed works (i.e. other paintings, videos, poetry pieces, etc.). And it is very important to ask questions here. This way it is not just about you as the facilitator giving information but it is an exchange of information. For example, we are going to create a shadow puppet show based on journeys. In this section I may put: talk about journeys and voyages, what is the farthest you have gone from home? Where did you go? What was it like? Who has ever had a dream about going on a trip somewhere? Where was it? Talk about how we can show journeys in different forms from storytelling to film. Discuss Balinese shadow puppetry and storytelling, how epic narratives and historical stories are told through shadow imagery. Who has ever made shadows with their hands? Did they ever know someone who told great stories? Explain how we are going to create a story together and then represent it in shadow form. In order to run a successful workshop there needs to be a degree of enthusiasm on your part as the facilitator – you need to sell the project!

Step-by-step breakdown of activities:
Now break down exactly what happens step-by-step. As abilities in a group setting often vary it is useful to give yourself space to allow things to take longer than expected. With that said, patients often work diligently and enjoy deadlines and meeting them, but the process should be fun and stress-free. Instead of a day by day, I find it more useful to produce a step-by-step guide. This can be bullet points if its easier but should include: <ul><li>how you introduce the project</li><li>what are the materials used</li><li>what the first step is</li><li>how much time you expect the group to take to create the work</li><li>what the expected outcome is</li><li>having extra tasks for those who finish earlier so they are still involved</li><li>giving a moment towards the end where the group can reflect on the work made, perhaps each individual can share their work to the group (acknowledgement of the effort is key)</li><li>an exhibition of the work to share with staff, carers, friends and family.</li></ul>

> **Concluding activity:**
>
> Every project you do needs a concluding activity; though this is listed in the breakdown, it should be expanded here in its own section. It is important that the investment in the production of a work is acknowledged and treated as a success, for no matter the result it is a success. This activity can vary depending on the group and the dynamic. It can be a discussion about our favourite weather and how this was represented in the Haikus we wrote, or it can be a moment where each person holds up their painting to the rest of the group and receives acknowledgement and accolade, or it can be an exhibition where the works are framed, people are invited and tea and biscuits are served as if it were an opening in the world's best gallery – the work should always be treated as such and celebrated. An important dynamic of sharing will have been created and closing the workshop is central to the process of running it successfully.

> This last section of celebration of the work is very important. The most successful projects are the ones that reach a conclusion and have a presentation. This is because the idea of legacy is central to engaging in a creative practice at the end of our lives. This last artefact, be it a poem, a painting, a sculpture or photographs of a performance, often becomes the final tangible item an individual makes before death. To leave something behind becomes important not only for patients but for family as well. And of course most of the patients may not have artistic skill or practice, and struggle to complete the work. Yet with patience, bringing the work to completion and then celebrating that task gives the work itself a focus of appreciation that goes beyond just a simple surface aesthetic value. Time should be spent in the presentation of the work: framing paintings (matt board will suffice), editing a video and adding titles and music, setting up a performance and rehearsing the presentation, all bring a finished quality to the production. There should be no pressure to create an extraordinary event; simply this is a celebration of a task well done. Formalise it with an invitation sent out in advance, a poster, and prepare for the day with juice and snacks. Give the presentation the feel of a celebration, after all it is one. To offer a patient at the end of their lives a moment to feel proud and accomplished adds a dimension to the workshop that extends beyond the walls of the room where the practical work may take place.

Implementing a project: making it work

Though there may be supplies ordered and a project plan completed, the reality of implementing a project may differ from our expectations and I have found that we should always be open for adaptation and change as the project unfolds. At times I found complex projects needing to be scaled down to be more accessible and at other times I found simple projects to lack the energy and drive needed to sustain people's attention. Part of the work requires flexibility and creativity so that the approach of the facilitator is always patient-centred. It is important to put aside artistic ego, and though this seems obvious, at times our own need to create a beautiful work with patients can be strong. But identifying the difference between the results we are seeking and the results the participants are seeking is key to a successful negotiation. Anthropologist W.H. Goodenough gives an excellent practical approach, which he terms 'other-oriented' (Goodenough 1966, p.543). According to Goodenough, being other-oriented signifies a recognition of others where we become less ethnocentric, for it is easier for an individual to identify with a group than a group with an individual. Art critic and theorist Grant Kester expands on this notion, terming it 'empathetic identification' which requires 'active listening' (Kester 2004). This ability to listen allows greater collaboration instead of arriving at the workshop with a pre-formed and fixed vision of a final product.

What I found running my own groups was that in actuality there was very little difference in the tools and systems I engaged with as an artist in the hospice setting or in any other setting. I had a skill as a visual artist and I was in a position to share that skill with others. The basic pedagogical techniques of asking questions, giving praise, working individually, encouraging the group and allowing space for critical reflection were all valid and useful during the workshop. There were at times resistance to new forms. I discovered that bringing in a new creative approach can meet resistance, especially when it becomes about insecurity regarding virtuosity. I found one of the important things to encourage was that the process would be simple and straightforward and produce good results. If as a workshop facilitator you hold this perspective certain, it undoubtedly encourages the participants. And remember this is the case, for what the patients produce at whatever level of ability they have is worthy, and with the crafting hand of the artist it is easy to present a final product in a special way.

There may be times that there is resistance by some members of the group to participate while others are eager. This is also part of the process and should never be seen as an affront to the group or the facilitator. If possible individuals can work on their own separate projects in the room, or they can observe. What I found was that often by the second week those who resisted the new material and wanted to continue their own individual basic crafts projects would soon want to join the group project. An allowance needs to be made for patients like this who may enter into the project late. Due to their varying medical needs many patients come in and out of a group, but by no means should the main project stall due to this. It needs to be possible for a patient to prioritise their own care plan. This might mean seeing their nurse or physiotherapist before coming to a group, which will help them alleviate any worries they have about their physical illness in order to focus more successfully on working with the arts. Consistency is important – a patient who helped set up a still life for a photography project and then comes back to the workshop after a three-week recovery should still feel that they are part of the group and want to share in the results. So work must be kept rolling, allowing this entrance and exit of participants. Generally there is always a core of participants who become involved and driven to see the project to completion. After all a sense of deadline becomes heightened for obvious reasons in end of life care, and finishing a project can often become an imperative.

Working within the frameworks of institutions
Case study: creating art together
The first patient I worked with was on a one to one basis, referred by a community nurse. Joyce was in her early fifties and in the late stages of motor neuron disease (MND). She could no longer control the brush or speak. I held the brush in her hand and spoke through the process with her. Her head hung to one side from which she could still move her eyes to follow the brush. I had not heard of MND before and was unaware of what physically was happening to Joyce. Nevertheless we were able to communicate, and though she could not speak or move more than her eyes from me to the page, her hoarse laugh was contagious and uplifting. We made jokes about the tree, added some apples to pick later for lunch and for that first hour that we met, connected through a language that was not based in words. The results of the painting were lovely, and though I had moved her hand with the brush, it felt very much Joyce's own work.

This first encounter has always stayed with me for it made me realise the power of collaboration, patience, listening and how creative arts work could be beneficial in this area.

Working in partnership with other institutions

Part of my work at St Christopher's has been placements in various other institutions to run workshops as part of the wider work of both the team of artists and the hospice itself. I have worked in care homes, nursing homes, rehabilitation centres and other hospices both for adults and children. These arts projects have all been part of an expanding hospice responsibility to support older people, those living with non-malignant disease and teenagers moving through transition from children to adult services. Working with other local adult hospices has also helped to create new and existing partnerships through utilising the creative arts. I always find it interesting how the arts could support the hospice's wider strategic vision to take the services it offered to ever wider groups of people. Though I have a variety of artistic skills, they are of course limited to my training and interests and thus my own projects are always a reflection of that.

My first external arts project was in a neurological rehabilitation centre with a group that had an age range from 19 to 70 years. Many of the patients had little to no motor skills, and running the group project required the assistance of nurses and nursing assistants. An important recommendation about working with a combination of nurses, carers and patients is that the workshop is actually benefitting everyone present. Though the practical work is aimed at engaging the patients, I have found that the experience can often affect those who come to assist. As an arts group facilitator it is important to integrate all participants who are in the workshop and to be upfront and open about a philosophy of inclusion. Many support staff will complete the work for the patient and dismiss their abilities. This is less about negligence than about a lack of patience with the artistic process. If you have arrived at a place of feeling comfortable enough in your creative field to run a workshop then you know that it takes dedication, practice and patience to have achieved your skill set. The same needs to be reinforced to support staff so that they too enjoy the process. Especially when running a group and, in reality, being a guest within their institution, there is a fine line in implementing your own creative approach and working within the existing culture. Each institution has varying protocols and modes of management which will affect the way the workshop is developed. I have discovered that often, the hardest resistance to new forms of creative expression will come from staff not patients. Even if support staff insist patients are not interested or incapable, our role as community artists is to give the patient an opportunity and to believe that everyone has a capability. This is what counts in the end. I have also learned from experience that patients can become so accustomed to being managed that a change in dynamic can actually reawaken their energy and re-engage their intellect.

Case study: the power of the creative process

Betty was a patient in the frail and elderly ward of a care home I was running a project in. Though she seemed despondent at first she slowly integrated week after week in the group project. The nurses would sometimes not bring Betty to the group, but I often insisted she attended regardless. By the end of my placement there we had created a series of bold artworks with the residents. My exhibition took place in the canteen, where the manager had agreed I could hang the works. Decorating the living space with patients' artwork enlivens the room and reminds all those who are there that these are individuals with active imaginations and sets of skills. When Betty's son came to the exhibition he sought me out to tell me that he was amazed to see how week to week his mother had changed. He had been visiting her for a long time but never had he actually seen her progress. For the first time she not only seemed to engage more physically but mentally she was more alert. He was overjoyed because she had written a letter to her estranged sister, which was long overdue. Betty's engagement in the creative process and with the group allowed her to also engage in her own personal reflections at the end of her life.

Understanding the power of the creative arts, even when there may be resistance to change in an institution, is important. It gives the certainty that what we are doing matters, and to not give up when it seems that obstacles are placed in our way.

Working alongside other health care professionals

The time spent developing a creative practice allows the participants moments of reflection on their situation, and as such gives them an opportunity to socialise and discuss these reflections. This gives the artist a degree of responsibility with information which may be disclosed during group settings, regarding health issues or emotional needs. Another important factor when getting started is to be aware of the wider network of care that is taking place. The arts are one of many factors contributing to the wellbeing of the patient. Though the logistics of planning and delivering projects are important, it should be noted that this is part of a larger system which is in place. The creation of a space in the workshop means that patients at times may feel comfortable with disclosing sensitive information regarding either their physical or emotional state. Alternately it can be that the workshop is the most active part of their routine and as such we are able to witness some struggles or challenges that the patient is going through either emotionally or physically. This is why a referral system is often important. At St Christopher's, artists and arts therapists regularly meet with a larger staff body that includes nurses, physiotherapists, social workers and chaplains to exchange information on specific patients and their families and carers. This is an opportunity to flag concerns, note observations across different fields and to offer different modes of support. Though the organisation of St Christopher's may be more complex than smaller institutions, there is always someone acting as a key worker, normally a senior nurse or a social worker. This ensures that any needs or issues that you become aware of are put into a wider system of care and service for the benefit of the multi-disciplinary team, but more importantly the patient.

Two important challenges

I have experienced that working in end of life care has both its rewards and challenges. To become a central figure in someone's life at the end of their life is an important role that can really engage us emotionally. But in addition to this I would cite two other important challenges to the newcomer working in arts and health care in this setting:

1. Our own argument for limitations. By this I mean, as a creative arts practitioner we can often doubt ourselves, both as artists and as facilitators. When we do this we can often convince ourselves that we are not capable of pulling off a larger more complex project with a group of patients. It is important to recognise when we ourselves are placing limitations on what may be, in reality, picked up from participants in the workshop experience. I have found that thinking big, and outside of the box, has brought me the most rewarding experiences I have ever had in creating arts projects. When I succumbed to my own arguments limiting the project scope, either through fear of failure or laziness to put in the effort, I ended up with

repetitive arts projects that were not as engaging or productive as my other efforts.

2. Always go with your intention and be confident of your skill if you find yourself challenged by other staff who do not think the participants are capable of engaging. Though with very good intentions, I sometimes find that carers and nurses could be very resistant to new forms of art making. As a community artist, I brought forth my expertise and knowledge to the task at hand. This made me the expert in that field, and as such I can create a valid argument with reluctant nursing staff and volunteers why it is essential that the group, for example, build a totem pole in the garden. This requires a level of confidence where you take the risk to truly believe in yourself and your abilities and therefore the abilities of those you are working with.

Changing culture

Case study: a surprising encounter

In one care home I created a documentary project alongside our art groups. One of the participants was a Middle Eastern woman in her forties who had suffered a stroke and had limited mobility and I was told that she could not speak. I would ask her questions during the workshop and the carers would speak over her, either answering for her or continually telling me that she could not speak and furthermore she could not speak English. One session I was teaching another patient how to use the video camera and we were filming her. I asked the resident where she was from, and in quite plain English, in a very low tone she answered 'I am from Pakistan.' I was stunned and continued interviewing her, though the rest of her answers were difficult to understand, her interview made it to the documentary for all to see that not only could she communicate, she could also speak English and happily engage in a documentary interview.

Stories like this are countless, and are an important part of engaging in the arts in end of life care and its related settings. Much of the work is about changing the culture within institutions which are unaccustomed to the power of the arts to transform and to express. In order to be an agent of change with the tools to engage both patients, staff, friends and family it is important to find the correct combination of being self-assured and being a good listener. This way each project can be fine tuned to the institutional setting in which you may find yourself. There is no one basic model of implementation because the dynamics between people that are created in any work environment shift from location to location. But what can be systematised is your own approach: how you deal with set-backs, how you learn to be flexible with the delivery of the project, and how you maintain the perseverance to see a workshop through to its end complete with a celebratory event, no matter how small.

When asked by staff why I may be offering to produce a radio theatre play with a group of people in one institution instead of their expected 'macaroni collages' which I learned they had been doing for a number of years, I explained that my specialty as an artist is to create collaborative works and that the participants had suggested the theme themselves. I also explained that I had brought new materials to engage the patients (microphones, instruments for making sound effects) and that the work is about memory and nostalgia, recalling the old radio shows of their youth. As I had already planned out the workshop, I shared this plan, and used it as a way to speak through the process so it was clear. Once staff saw that there was a structure and a plan which had been instigated by those involved, as well as materials and the enthusiasm, they were more comfortable to help bring the project to completion.

My time working at St Christopher's has exposed me to a variety of clinic settings, health care professionals, and patients from all walks of life. I have learned an incredible amount about the city of London, through a continual flow of memory data shared from patients who have lived in the area all of their lives, or who migrated here as part of their story. This has helped me create a tangible picture of the metropolis from post-war to present. Through time my projects have become more involved and interesting as I incorporate new ideas, listen for input from patients and staff on improving the workshops, and bring in inspiration from various sources of outside cultural activities I attend and engage with. As artists we are influenced by the myriad of resources and material that we can bring to devising new projects. Working with patients and carers facing the end of life and being open to these sources of inspiration and incorporating them into the way I create our work with patients has allowed me a continual flow of fresh ideas. After all, in many ways, creating artworks in such settings has as much to do with celebrating life and living as it does to do with death and dying.

Reflection

The experiences that we carry with us of the process of deciding to apply for a new job, completing an application form and being successfully interviewed can often establish the foundations from which our work will grow and develop within a new organisation as well as create and determine our future professional identity.

We must not underestimate the importance of filling out job application forms effectively and the seriousness of impeccable planning ahead of a formal interview process. Writing a personal statement or a passage as part of an application form on why you want the job and why you want to work for the particular organisation requires careful crafting and consideration. I always think it is sensible to ask someone you know well to read through your application form before submitting it. Filling out information regarding education, qualification and experience should be straightforward enough. However, any free text gives you the opportunity to put forward your strengths and show your personality, which, quite apart from ticking the boxes regarding any formal requirements, might also be an important aspect of the form that enables you to progress forward to an interview stage.

One of the central subjects that we read about during Roberto's sharing of his experiences and his knowledge of the practicalities of starting out working in end of life care is that of planning well. Whether it is for an interview, or putting together a coherent proposal for an arts project to be carried out within a particular setting, Roberto instils within us the essential need to be prepared. Writing a project proposal, such as that given to us by Roberto as an example, is not only for the benefit of ourselves as artists or therapists. As we hear from him, such plans and proposals can be used to convince both those who are going to be actively involved in the work as well as those staff who might feel disinclined to motivate patients and others to move out of the norm and try something new and different. Honing and utilising the skills and craft of persuasion are important elements of the job of providing a service such as the creative arts, the benefits of which to many might be confused and unclear. Where people have used and experienced the creative arts as part of their setting previously, they may equally have become repetitive or stuck and ceased to be dynamic or beneficial interventions (Hartley and Payne 2008).

Roberto talks eloquently about his experience of being interviewed for a community artist position at St Christopher's Hospice. On the whole, he prepares well, looking at the website and researching into the history and service development of the hospice movement. He also knows himself well enough to understand that he communicates effectively and can remain relaxed during stressful situations. This knowledge and confidence will serve him well when he is asked to respond to an unexpected, yet crucial, question: 'Tell us about your relationship with death and dying.' Here we touch upon an extremely relevant matter. Our own fears, concerns and previous experiences of death and dying will colour and affect our relationships with dying people, bereaved relatives and friends, as well as the relationships we have with the colleagues we work alongside and the organisations that we and they work as part of. It is therefore important that we consider our relationship with death and dying seriously and take some time to understand it. Roberto brings this matter full circle when he ends his writing with highlighting for us that 'creating artworks in such settings has as much to do with celebrating life and living as it does to do with death and dying'. However, we must not misunderstand this. There is a common misconception that hospices sometimes collude with an unspoken denial of the very thing they are set up to address (Randall and Downie 2006). We must strive to become comfortable enough with our own relationship with death so that this does not become a reality. What Roberto really means here is that when death and dying are accorded their proper place, acknowledged, accepted and understood as part of life and living, our experience of using the arts as part of the dying process can lead those people who are experiencing it to a heightened sense of life and their place within it.

References

Goodenough, W. H. (1966) *Cooperation in Change: An Anthropological Approach to Community Development.* New York: John Wiley & Sons.

Hartley, N. and Payne, M. (2008) *The Creative Arts in Palliative Care.* London and Philadelphia, PA: Jessica Kingsley Publishers.

Kester, G.H. (2004) *Conversation Pieces: Community + Communication in Modern Art.* Berkeley and Los Angeles, CA, London: University of California Press.

Randall, F. and Downie, R. (2006) *The Philosophy of Palliative Care – Critique and Reconstruction.* Oxford: Oxford University Press.

Chapter 10

Looking After Yourself

Marion Tasker and Nigel Hartley

Introduction

There is an assumption that those people working in end of life care need or deserve a lot of support and should take extra care to look after themselves. We know that the way that some end of life care practitioners have portrayed working with the dying over the years may have supplemented the belief that this is so (De Hennezel 1999; Hartley 2001; Lee 1996; Renzenbrink 2011). However, it is of course true that working with people who are dying and supporting those people who are bereaved presents us with certain personal and professional challenges which need to be addressed in order to sustain good professional practice and a healthy outlook on life.

We have already touched on the area of coping with working in end of life care in Chapter 8 'Bereavement and Loss'. Many people consistently ask those of us who work in this area how we manage to do so on a day to day basis. There does seem to be an endless fascination from many about what it is like to be consistently working with the dying and the bereaved, and how professionals who do so survive in the long term. In many ways this is understandable, due to the inherent fear about death and the dying process which we witness as part of the everyday life of most individuals and the communities within which they live. However, with regard to working in end of life care, there is no straightforward answer to this question other than to perhaps put it into a broader context and to open up the enquiry in the following way: 'How does each one of us cope doing the work that we do, whether it be in end of life care, working in a bank, or running the country?'

In this chapter, we hear from Marion, who is an experienced community artist who works at St Christopher's Hospice. Following an introduction and sharing some personal information, Marion goes on to address the area of looking after yourself when working in end of life care, and she covers the following areas:

- Working in an unfamiliar territory

- Working with the dying

- Finding appropriate support

- Utilising existing support systems and structures

- Formal supervision and support

- Informal supervision and support

- Developing self-awareness

- Annual appraisals

- Continuing professional development (CPD)

- Boundaries

- When things get personal

- Understanding our own relationship to death, dying and loss

- Recognising and coping with stress.

Marion adds in a number of short stories to highlight some of the points raised, and the chapter ends with my thoughts and reflections.

Marion: my background

My name is Marion Tasker and I knew as a child that I wanted to be an artist. In fact, rather precociously, I wrote my autobiography at the age of eight that confirmed this aspiration. On leaving school I studied a vocational course at college for three years which covered technical and botanical illustration. When I graduated, I worked for a medical publishers in London where I was employed as a medical illustrator and then, a few years later, went on to manage the illustration department. I began to accumulate private clients to the point that the transition from employment to being a freelance and self-employed medical illustrator was a natural one. I worked both from home and at several West End design studios. At this time my ambition was to earn as much money as possible and I had an aspiration to eventually bring together a group of artists and designers to form a small business. Both the work that hospices do and the arts therapies were completely unknown to me. It was purely through a chance conversation with a neighbour who worked at St Christopher's Hospice that I learned about the work that they did and I decided to apply to become a volunteer for the organisation. My interest was to volunteer on the inpatient wards helping with general practical duties, but when I was interviewed, they were keen to utilise my art skills and I agreed to help out by supporting a paid artist in one of the regular art groups which were organised for patients and family members.

This experience was to change the direction of my career and I now work full time as a community artist and have recently completed a counselling degree. I am part of a team of artists that comprises arts therapists as well as community artists.

Working in an unfamiliar territory

When I first stepped through the doors of St Christopher's Hospice I understandably felt nervous and anxious about how I should be, what I should say, and what I might be in danger of doing wrong. What I might see and how I would be seen were things that I found myself both worrying and fantasising about.

Early on when I began working as a community artist I had an experience of saying the wrong thing to a patient. Although embarrassing, the encounter was a learning experience and concluded with the patient and myself laughing together.

Case study: faux pas

A patient who generally attended the morning art group I was running felt ill on this particular day and declined the offer to come along to the group. I immediately suggested that she stay where she was and 'rest in peace'. As soon as the words came out of my mouth I cringed. The patient's response was that maybe that this was not the best thing to say, and then burst into laughter.

I spoke to my manager about this, and realised, of course, that most professionals working in end of life care have similar experiences from time to time. This incident and my manager's response to it helped me, as I realised that as long as what I said and did was not ill intended and I could learn from it, most people would understand. I also learned that whatever is going in in people's lives, even if they are in the last stages of life, they are still a person with a mix of emotions and experiences, sometimes sad and distressed, and sometimes humorous and playful.

I also realise that people, just because they are dying, are not saints. There is a tendency to patronise and overprotect the dying. I have learned that they are still human beings, just like myself, who can be provocative, abrupt, angry and challenging. As well as the many other human characteristics we all display from time to time, it is probable that we will continue to utilise all of these characteristics until we die. So for me, I have discovered that the challenge is not just in how I relate to other people, but also how I learn to respond to them relating to me.

Case study: being told where to go!

A patient who was bed-bound on the ward had been referred to me for art. The patient had Parkinson's disease and was finding it difficult to communicate. The nursing staff had assured me that it was a good idea to go and talk to him about doing some art. I went into his room full of enthusiasm, suggesting the idea that he might like to do some painting. Encouraged by the fact that he was trying to say something to me I moved closer to him and listened intently trying to decipher what he was saying. In a sudden burst of energy he told me quite succinctly what he thought about my idea and where to go. I left the room.

I felt completely wounded by this response and the memory of it has stayed with me to this day. It tapped into all kinds of personal insecurities. On one hand, I came away feeling nervous about approaching any other new patients who would be referred to me. On another, I have learned the importance of planning before I go to visit a new patient. I now read patient notes before meeting them as well as having, where possible, a handover discussion with the referrer or other member of staff. This is so that I can get a sense of the person who I am about to meet in advance. However, there is a down side of this. In getting information in advance, I feel that we can potentially make assumptions about the people we are about to meet and this could get in the way of making a successful relationship and therefore damage the possibility of working effectively together.

Whenever I encounter such difficult situations, as even with experience I find that I still have complicated encounters with patients from time to time, I tell someone about them. I seek out my manager, or a colleague to talk them through, and this has proved to be invaluable. I have learned that if we feel we have done or said the wrong thing to a patient, it pays dividends to talk to someone I work alongside about it. In this way, I can get support to put things right, whether to put things right practically or to put things right in my own mind. If we share a problem, we can get support. If we keep it to ourselves, the potential is for it to get bigger and out of control.

My early experiences of working at the hospice have been steps along the road to acknowledging the need to look after myself. I always think that working with dying people is the kind of work that might be described as being on the 'coal face'. It can be raw and brutal, but it can also be creative and inspiring. I find that the beauty of it is that it is never mundane and very rarely predictable.

Many of my fellow artists who work at the hospice are trained as arts therapists, and other community artists have other qualifications in counselling or psychology. A few years back, I decided to embark on a degree course in person-centred counselling in order to gain new insights and to understand more fully the work that I was doing. I have found doing this has been invaluable and has helped to support my work with patients and family members at the hospice. It has enabled me to be able to stand back from the work I do and to develop my self-awareness in order to notice and reflect more thoughtfully on what happens within my encounters with patients on a day to day basis.

It is clear to me that deciding to undertake a counselling degree was a way of discovering a new kind of support for myself. It is important to remember that the choices we all make in finding ways to support and sustain the work that we do will be highly individual. In sharing some of my experiences, I am hoping that they might resonate with those working in similar fields and enable us all to think a little more about supporting ourselves as we consistently work in an environment where we are predominantly reflecting about the patients and family members with whom we work.

Working with the dying

The artists who work at St Christopher's do so in a variety of different settings. They run groups at the hospice and as part of outreach projects in care homes and GP practices within the catchment area. They work individually with patients and family members both in the hospice and within their own homes. They talk to and teach a range of professionals about the work that they do. They also support the hospices' public education and health promotion programme by running a range of arts groups with patients, family members, carers, other staff, volunteers, and also members of the general public.

As you can imagine, working as part of each of these very different scenarios brings individual challenges and stressors; however, I find that there is always a feeling of accomplishment and success.

Despite mentioning that I ended up working at St Christopher's by accident and had no overt desire to work with patients at the end of their lives, I can remember as a teenager that I did, in fact, have an interest in helping others and at one point I thought that I might work abroad for a non-governmental organisation (NGO). The need or wish to care for others and to do something that would make a difference was clearly there. The different ways that we end up doing the work that we do within the caring professions will be varied and while, for some people, they will have been introduced to caring for frail or ill family members from an early age, for others, like myself, they will have stumbled across the opportunity more by accident in order to fulfil a need in themselves. I find that it is fine, even essential, to acknowledge that as we work in the caring professions, many of us will have a personal investment in the work we do.

Finding appropriate support

My experience of working in end of life care has taught me that, first and foremost, it is the responsibility of the individual to recognise the need for different kinds of support. Hospices, in particular, offer robust support and supervision structures. Regular supervision meeting with an experienced manager or organised support groups with peers led by an external supervisor are commonplace. However, although managerial supervision is normally mandatory, attendance at support groups is often not, and I find it strange how many staff choose not to attend such meetings. Most of us will prefer support in different ways, and it is conceivable that attending support groups with peers, for some, will not be something that they choose to engage in. Self-care can sometimes be a contentious issue between employer and employee. Supervision and support is written about extensively by professionals within the fields of psychology and counselling (Renzenbrink 2004), but little is written for those people working outside of these fields.

There can be a contradiction here between the professional's way of attending to issues of support and supervision and that of the employer. This can sometimes jar with an organisational approach, where there is an obvious need for the employee to develop a robust and resilient outlook and to be able to get on with the job. After all, the organisation can only offer so many support and supervision structures, and beyond these, a responsibility must lie with the professional to find individual ways of supporting themselves.

How successful people who work in end of life care are at discovering their own ways of being supported might be something to question. Some data appears to demonstrate that, particularly in end of life care, there are high levels of time off taken by staff who are depressed, and absenteeism from work may be extensive. These statistics can also be seen in other areas of the caring professions too, such as medicine and nursing. This illustrates clearly the importance of how an organisation persuades staff to utilise the support and supervision structures which it offers, in order to sustain good mental and physical health among employees. I often ask myself, what makes us resilient in this work? Probably, as Weisman suggests, that good copers seek and use resources of all kinds (1979), and having the ability to source our own support systems and to be creative in doing so holds part of the answer to this question. I have found that having good supportive family networks and groups of friends, as well as a range of hobbies and activities outside of the workplace pays dividends for a consistently good state of mind. For instance, I have a motorbike, and love nothing more than going out biking with my friends. I find that such an activity inspires and renews me in ways that I find impossible to articulate.

Utilising existing support systems and structures

Our first point of call, when thinking about support and supervision for the work that we do therefore, should be to discover what mechanisms the organisation for which we work have put into place for our wellbeing. For example, at St Christopher's, as well as individual managerial supervision, regular team meetings, and the possibility of attending a peer support group with an outside facilitator, there are also more informal sessions available for staff such as yoga or massage. I have discovered, through working alongside many people who do this work, that for some, however much support and supervision will be on offer from the organisation, they will never feel that it is enough. I feel it is sometimes too easy to blame the organisation which we work for, when we feel that support and supervision is not what we think it should be. This is an interesting issue, and I often wonder why, for some people, this is so. I have learned that support and supervision within the work place need to be utilised to the best advantage. What I mean by this, is that planned, organised support needs planning and organisation from those who need to use it. For example, I find it useful to know that a support group is coming up, as I can plan the kinds of things I need to talk about in advance; the same goes for my planned managerial supervision sessions. If something happens with a patient, or a group that I am running, which I need to talk through, if a support group is planned in two days' time, I am able to feel supported through knowing that there will be a chance to unpack the issue in the not too distant future. However, occasionally, something happens where I need to talk something through immediately. I am fortunate that my manager is always happy to give me some time as the need arises, and, of course, we must not forget how lucky we are, particularly within hospices, to be able to talk to our peers in a more informal way on a daily basis. Going back to the people who never feel as if enough support is on offer, I worry that they may get easily overwhelmed with the work they are doing, and maybe these are the ones who are more likely to take more time off work in order to recuperate. I also wonder if these people do not have healthy support mechanisms in place within their lives outside of the work place?

The question remains, what is enough when we are talking about support and supervision for end of life care practitioners? Renzenbrink (2011) talks about 'relentless self-care' for those people who work with the dying. Although this is understandable, only a proportion of the responsibility for support and supervision should lie with the employer. As trained professionals, we should realise the importance of self-support and we must learn to discover the unique ways that we may need to achieve this for ourselves. This might include some external private supervision, as outlined, as a necessity during some professional training programmes, or something as simple as meditating, exercising, enjoying being with family members, or biking with friends, as in my own case.

While in some working environments we may go home and talk to our families and friends about the day we have had or things we have found difficult, this is the same in any job, and I find that this can be useful and supportive. However, when working with people who are particularly vulnerable, the issue of confidentiality is an important one to remember, and although I find it helpful to talk generally about my work with family and friends, it is important to remember that to talk about the detail is not appropriate.

Confidentiality is something we need to be conscious of in all of our communication outside of the workplace, as it is not appropriate explicitly to talk about a patient or their family members or carers, to friends and family.

Formal supervision and support

One of the issues of working part time within an end of life care organisation, is that, although monthly support and supervision groups are organised and offered to all staff, the time of the day or week when they are offered might be such that it is not possible to attend. There are other options, however, and my own experience has shown me that it is important, when working within the therapeutic, supportive professions, that we look for a personal supervisor. This will be someone outside of the organisation, and, although possible, it is unlikely that this will be paid for by your workplace. This can therefore be costly, although I have found that the benefits certainly warrant the cost. It will be important to remember that if you are making a bid for funding, for a substantive arts or arts therapies post within a hospice, or for a more specific time-limited project, adding any formal support and supervision costs into the proposal might be important.

Supervision can take different forms and sometimes, there can be a difference between clinical supervision and managerial supervision. In simple terms *managerial supervision* might be described as a pragmatic look at the work you are doing. It would usually be facilitated by your line manager within the organisation in which you work. It might be an informal weekly or monthly catch up with your manager. Things discussed might be goals of the organisation, training expectations, manual handling, fire training or diversity training. The amount of work you are involved in might be focussed on and any performance-related issues would be discussed here too. There should also be an opportunity to discuss any targets and future new projects. Although more focussed on management, we must not forget that our managers will, on the whole, be experienced practitioners in end of life care and the style of supervision and support we get from them is open to negotiation. It should be entirely possible to talk through any issues regarding your clinical work, and I always think it is important to agree with your manager that this will be possible. It is well worth utilising their experience to get the help and support you need, and, in my experience, managers are usually more than willing to offer this.

Formal clinical support or supervision might often be facilitated by someone outside the organisation or from a different department within the organisation. This is an opportunity to bring any issues regarding your work with patients and families to be discussed within a closed environment. It might also be an opportunity to talk about any issues with colleagues or management that may have arisen in a confidential manner. Many organisations, such as St Christopher's, will offer this opportunity on a regular basis to all staff who work with patients and families. It is my experience that often, people who have had therapeutic training of some kind will seek out more personal formal supervision from a supervisor who follows a similar approach to their own practice, outside of the organisation. For instance, when I did my degree in person-centred counselling, I sought a supervisor who followed that approach. This support enabled me to keep in touch with my training and to also witness the practice of the approach in action during the supervision session, so I was also able to link theory to practice. It is also possible, if you feel that it is needed, to join a supervision group external to the organisation. I have found that there can be huge benefits doing this, especially where there are people from different schools of thought. The learning and support can be great, both stimulating and challenging. However, it is important to remember that arranging your own external formal, clinical supervision can be financially costly, and it is useful to factor this into your monthly spending.

St Christopher's currently offers the following support and supervision to all staff including artists and arts therapists:

- regular 1–1 supervision meetings with the manager or senior practitioner in their department

- senior practitioners meet weekly for 1–1 supervision with their manager

- all teams have access to monthly group meetings with their manager to reflect on practice and discuss case studies

- monthly clinical supervision groups are available to all staff who work with patients and families and these groups are facilitated by an external professional.

Informal supervision and support

As part of my training as a counsellor, I have been taught that I should be in formal supervision when I am practising. I am also required to be in formal clinical supervision in order to be registered to practise with the relevant professional body. For some people who work as artists within health care institutions it might not be a either a professional imperative or requirement to seek regular formal supervision or support. However, there are other ways of finding less formal support mechanisms. One of the most useful ways to access informal support and supervision, as I have already mentioned, is from your peers and colleagues. I have discovered that this is, by far, the most useful and best resource we have. I feel that I am fortunate that I work alongside a large group of artists and therapists, all of whom have specific qualities and skills which can be useful when seeking out informal support or supervision. I find that we work well together. We have a mutual trust, honesty and respect conducive to the sharing of the challenges and difficulties that we discover in our work without fear, judgement or ridicule. It is also important to share our triumphs and accomplishments together with our colleagues, as this too can lead to a sense of being supported and acknowledged for the things we have achieved both with and for the patients and families who we offer our services to.

Working in a hospice or other end of life care organisation, we must keep in mind how fortunate we are to work alongside other people as part of a dedicated team. Working as part of this team, we should use the resources for informal support and supervision that are available to us. My experience shows that the very nature of seeking support from, and sharing my work with, other team members can be both bonding and also enhance working relationships.

If you are the only artist or therapist working in an organisation it will be useful to identify at least one colleague who you might be able to talk with informally every now and again. Also remember that support of this kind should be mutual and you should also offer to listen to the issues of, and offer support to, your colleague as part of the process.

It also might be an idea to get together with a group of like-minded colleagues from time to time to benefit from some peer support or discussion in a group. This can easily take place over lunch, and can offer another way to support and educate each other about the work you do. Myself and the other artists and therapists I work with do this from time to time. We also offer half-day workshops, which includes time for support and supervision to groups of artists and activity co-ordinators who work in end of life care or within local care homes. People who attend these workshops have embraced and acknowledged the value of being able to support and learn from each other and the importance of keeping in contact with people facing similar challenges in their own workplace and to take time to learn about the different ways in which problems have been acknowledged and addressed.

Developing self-awareness

I find that an important question to ask myself regularly is 'how well do I really know myself?' Michael Mayne talks of 'this intimate stranger I call me' (Mayne 2002). I have found that the continuing journey of getting to know myself can be as painful as it is rewarding, but I find that this particular journey enhances my understanding, not only of myself, but of myself in relationships to both others and the work that I do. Recognising behaviour patterns and responses does not necessarily denote a necessity to change but a necessity to take note and be mindful of how we impact those around us and also how the behaviour of others impacts us. As every experience we have in working with those who are facing death and dying is unique, so, I find, is my response to the situations I find myself in. Of course, with experience, I am learning ways of dealing with this, but from time to time, I still find my responses to certain people and things unexpected and surprising.

It is worth considering, although not a prerequisite of the work, having some kind of personal counselling or therapy at times. This might be something that a manager or supervisor might discuss with you and I can think of times when my supervisor has seen something in my response to a patient's situation and has suggested I might like to look at it within my own personal therapy. Personal counselling or therapy of some kind does not have to be on-going, but I find that it is useful to return to this kind of self-support when I need to focus more concretely on specific issues and events within my own life. When many of these things are instigated by the work that I am involved in on a day to day basis, I find that having a few therapy or counselling sessions can unlock some important issues and can also help to guard against over identification. There can be no question that for me, engaging in this kind of support from time to time can help me remain strong and grounded in the relationships that I form with patients, family members and carers.

Thic Nhat Hanh, Buddhist monk, teacher, author and poet says:

> ...to me, the practice of a healer, therapist, teacher, or any helping professional should be directed towards him or herself first, because if the helper is unhappy, he or she cannot help many people. We practice enjoying the positive elements in life in order to nourish the flower in us, and we practice in order to transform the seeds of suffering in us. Otherwise we cannot succeed in our work helping other people. (1991)

I constantly find his words helpful and reassuring.

Annual appraisals

Annual appraisal should be an aspect of managerial supervision offered by a professional health care organisation. Having been self-employed for many years I had never had an appraisal preceding my work at St Christopher's. I was a little nervous at the prospect. I imagined that it would be a review of my work and I worried that I would be judged and deemed unfit for not having achieved enough, or made enough difference, over the year. In actuality, the experience of this has been very different and I now embrace the opportunity to reflect on aspects of my work that I feel have gone well and those times when I feel that I have struggled due to a range of different factors. In the areas where I feel that I have struggled, it is useful to have the opportunity to go over these issues and to learn how I might have done things differently. On the other hand, maybe I am able to just acknowledge that something was difficult and I would not have been able do anything differently. I find that it is hugely reaffirming to talk about things that have gone well, and I always feel a sense of achievement being reminded of the positive experiences which have been too easy to put to the back of my mind and to forget about. I am always surprised by the extent of the work that has been done over the year. Often, on a day to day basis, I work through my schedule, and although pleased to have achieved the work that I set out to do, it is easy to move on quickly to the next thing. Projects begin and end, and exhibitions of work are hung and displayed. Having the opportunity to look back is affirming and can often act as a bedrock for the challenges that the following year might bring.

Continuing professional development (CPD)

Continuing professional development (CPD) is also important for our own development and self-care. It is normally brought up at an annual appraisal, and discussed regularly during managerial supervision. Those people who belong to a professional body will also be required to undergo a certain number of hours of CPD every year. This will include attending training days on relevant subjects, any formal educational programmes undertaken, and also, for some professionals, any training which is mandatory as part of professional re-registration. In reality, it may be difficult to fit such things into the working year, but it is a very important part of our own development and should be kept central to our day to day work. Not only is it important to keep up with new developments in the field within which you work, but it can also be an empowering way to look after yourself and to develop your own competency and confidence to continue working effectively. In renewing myself in this way, I have found that I can feel more confident and capable in delivering services to patients and family members. Many hospices will have their own education programme for staff, and it is important to be aware of this and to utilise it when needed. When I have attended workshops both at St Christopher's education centre and in other end of life care organisations I have felt inspired and motivated. Hearing about new ideas, new ways of looking at things, new perspectives and the chance to meet and hear other professionals talk about their experiences and share their own coping mechanisms can be very useful. Recently at St Christopher's education centre, we hosted the 2nd International Arts Symposium in end of life care. The two-day conference was rich and rewarding, and I met together with a large group of artists, therapists, nurses, social workers and other professionals, all of whom had a specific interest in the role of the arts in this area. I came away feeling nourished by the experience and ready to move forward with new ideas and a new energy. I also felt valued and acknowledged by the organisation that

I work for and also for the role I play within it. I find that even the smallest acknowledgment of work done and the success achieved can make a huge difference to how I feel.

Boundaries

I have found that maintaining professional boundaries can sometimes be challenging in end of life care. There are dynamics while working with someone who is dying that might not arise while working with someone who is not facing the end of their life. For the patients and family members, the differences between friendships and professional relationships can sometimes be confusing. We might feel the urgency to meet the needs that a patient or family member presents beyond that of our professional remit. We also know that one day, we will die too, and this very fact can often link us to our patients in ways that can appear unfathomable and can therefore change the very nature of the relationships that we form. It is these relationships that are integral to the work of the artist or therapist and I am constantly tested by their varied and complex nature.

I find that the development of social networking has also added another complicated dynamic which needs to be considered. This might not appear to be a common problem with, or consideration for, the older generation who we are working with, but as we begin to work with people more familiar with this way of communicating I believe it will be something that we need to consider regularly as part of our work. There can be no doubt that the development of digital media offers huge potential for using the arts and therapies to people when they are vulnerable and isolated. It becomes more common that many therapists and artists work via email and a variety of new computer programmes. With regard to the internet and social networking, however, two situations recently caused me to think about particular boundary issues.

Case study: 'friending'

A patient I had worked closely with one day requested me as a friend on a social network site. I felt quite shocked as suddenly I panicked that information about my personal life was, or would be available to patients and family members who I was working with. My way of dealing with this was to be honest and straightforward with the patient who had requested it, explaining that I kept my work separate from my personal life. The patient understood immediately.

Case study: my qualifications availability
I felt ill at ease when a client revealed that they had looked me up on the internet to find out about my professional credentials. Suddenly I felt quite exposed.

I thought very carefully about both of these situations. The social network incident, I felt, was quite straightforward to address and I was able to look at my privacy setting on my account and also decide whether in fact as a therapist it was appropriate for me to have a social network account at all. I decided to carry on with the account but to keep it under review, especially if another incident like this should happen.

The second incident I felt less able to control and, of course, anyone has the possibility to look anyone up on the internet. After I got over the initial surprise, I discussed it with my manager. We came to the conclusion that it was a natural response from a patient, and maybe something that we would both also do, should we want to know something more about a health care professional who was caring for us. Both reflecting on and discussing these situations helped me to process and to resolve them.

However, these experiences did make me realise and think about how much information is available to people on the internet. Personal information about ourselves is shared quite openly, often without our awareness, and this can indeed impact the relationships that we make both with patients and family members, especially if they look us up and discover personal information about us.

I often consider whether the boundaries of working as an arts or therapy practitioner within an end of life care institution should be set in stone or should they vary between the different patients and family members with whom we work?

The following two stories give brief examples of other times when I have needed to consider my responses to this question.

Case study: boundaries
I once had a holiday planned when I had just begun to work with a patient who clearly did not have much longer to live. As I was not going

away from home, my inclination was to come into work and meet with them during my leave.

I find that there is no right or wrong answer to this and sometimes I will come in to continue working with the patient and at other times I will not. Each situation is unique, and I find that I make the decisions based on a number of different factors which are exceptional to each situation. Early on in my working at the hospice I definitely found that I would invariably come in on my week off to work with patients, or to catch up with other things. Some of this was an ignorance of what the implications of this could be for my own self-care if done consistently over a period of time, and part of it was due to a previous freelance work ethic where set hours and days of work were quite alien because I was used to working according to deadlines set by the client. Now I am clearer about this I find that I think more carefully about each individual situation. I sometimes might try to see the patient just before I go on holiday and make sure that we have finished the work we are doing to a point that if the patient dies I would not feel as if there is something left uncompleted. In many ways, I often treat every art or therapy session I have with a patient as being the last. Although the work might not be completed fully, it does release me, in many ways, from feeling overly responsible. I often leave artwork with patients to continue working on when I am not around, and I often discover that even though the patient has died while I have been away, they have somehow found the necessary time and energy to complete the artwork.

Case study: phone number
A couple of times patients have asked for my personal phone number as a way of contacting me should they need to cancel an appointment.

This, in many ways, makes sense and can be completely understandable from a patient's perspective. I am often out of the office either running groups or doing home visits and it can be easy for me to miss a call and not realise an appointment has been cancelled. For artists and therapists, as with a range of other health care professionals, it is our personal responsibility to make sure that, as much as possible, we do not put ourselves at risk. In order to help with communication with patients and families, I keep an old mobile phone specifically for my work at the hospice. This can be particularly helpful when travelling around the community to visit patients at home. I do not store patients' personal numbers on it, and it is purely a telephone on which patients and family members can leave a message for me regarding appointments. I can also switch it off when I am not working. Chapter 7 gives some further useful information about policies and procedures for lone working in the community and the factors which need to be taken into account.

I have discovered that using the arts with patients and family members can enable us to reach a point of intimacy very quickly and this sometimes takes me by surprise. I have found that it is important to learn how to manage this on a day to day basis and I do not think that there is a blueprint. Securing our own personal and professional boundaries can be a way of maintaining a contained and protected place for the people we offer a service to, both to express and to explore the most difficult aspects of their dying process. Maintaining professional boundaries is also an integral part of our own self-care and of preserving our general wellbeing.

When things get personal

When working and living within the same geographical area there may come a time when a personal friend or family member will be in need of hospice or other end of life care services.

This happened to me a few years ago at St Christopher's and it raised some difficult and pertinent issues. It reminded me of how different it is to support people who are dying as a professional to supporting a personal friend or family member through the dying process. Below I share some notes from my personal journal written at this time.

Case study: 'a friend in the hospice'

I feel torn at times between wanting to be very present on the inpatient unit and sometimes not wanting to be around at all. I realise that I have ethical and professional responsibilities to consider too. I sometimes want to look up on the Electronic Patient Record (EPR) details of prognosis and treatment but I realise that this is not an option. I feel I am somehow managing the situation by concentrating and focussing on my role as a friend. I have spoken openly to her about my dilemmas and have come to an agreement about how I will support her through her illness and ultimately her death – about how I have to keep my professional role at the hospice separate and she seems to understand. She reminded me that she had previously worked as a volunteer at the hospice and so she does have some insight into the work we do and to the process and challenges of working alongside someone who is dying.

Although this was a complex situation, in many ways I found that I was very well supported by the nurses who cared for my friend on the ward. It made me realise how families and carers must feel when they are living alongside someone close who is dying, and how important the work of the professional team at the hospice really is. My friend died on Boxing Day that year and one of the nurses called me to tell me that she was close to dying to give me the opportunity to be with her. However, I had been out and I did not pick up the message until it was too late. I felt guilty that I could not be there with her. She had been frightened of dying. It would have been a chance for me to process what was happening and to say goodbye. Again, I am sure I experienced something of what family members, carers and friends go through routinely as part of someone's dying process.

In terms of caring for myself and supporting myself to move on from this experience, my friend was an artist and so I looked at some of her paintings and reflected on them. I wrote in my journal something about our friendship and I lit a candle in the Pilgrim Room which is a space within the hospice for reflection and memory. It was important for me to speak to the nurse who had been the person with her when she died. I found all of these things very reassuring. It was important for me to acknowledge this very personal loss and to give myself permission to grieve. I learned that grief, when managed and addressed, does not go on forever, and with some time-limited support I was able to move on with life in a normal and healthy way. I believe that such experiences are invaluable for us to develop both personally and professionally. Realising that grief is finite in such situations gives me a much better understanding and approach to the family members, carers and friends of those patients who are dying.

Understanding our own relationship to death, dying and loss

Part of understanding ourselves fully must include understanding our relationship to death, dying and loss. When we work on a daily basis with people who are dying or who are bereaved, understanding our relationship to death, dying and loss is important. This is because there will always be the possibility of certain feelings and responses being triggered as part of our work due to past experiences from within our personal lives.

Times when we have felt vulnerable, lonely, inadequate, powerless, out of control, unappreciated or abandoned may be picked up or reflected from certain patients and family members and our response can, in turn, affect how we respond to certain situations.

I am convinced that considering and understanding our relationship to death and our personal experiences of death and loss can help to make us more effective practitioners. A friend of mine who was training to become a priest was covering a module on bereavement as part of his course. He told me that he had never experienced the death of a close friend and the only family members who had died were his grandparents, who had died at what he described an expected age. He contemplated this and, in comparison to the other students on his course, who had all experienced different kinds of deaths, he had a feeling of inadequacy. He was clear that he needed to explore this in more depth, as it could indeed have an effect on his working with dying people following his ordination.

I am reminded personally of three close friends who died during my early twenties. I remember my other friends being the most important support during my period of grieving. We would sit together during the night in order to search out a meaning in death, and we created rituals in order to help us through the grieving process. Gradually we all moved on in different ways and I now look back and remember how informal it all was, and, how together, we were able to help each other through.

Recognising and coping with stress

One of the questions I was asked at my interview for the job of community artist at St Christopher's was how would I know if I was stressed and how would other members of staff recognise when I was stressed. You will have read more about interview processes and dealing with surprise questions in Chapter 9: 'Getting Started'. However, this was a question that particularly took me by surprise. As I was new to working in a caring profession, it was not something which I had considered in any depth and I felt that I answered the question somewhat flippantly. I said that people would know if I was stressed as when I was feeling under pressure I applied numerous layers of lipstick – the more stressed I become, another layer is applied.

Although a seemingly flippant response to the question, I believe that if such signals are acknowledged and understood, they can be a helpful way of triggering the need for some self-care or peer support. When talking to colleagues about how they recognise themselves to be stressed, their answers fall into a range of categories of stress symptom which were highlighted as part of a presentation given by Barbara Monroe in 2004:

- irritability

- depression

- loss of self-esteem

- over-involvement in work

- sleep disturbance

- weight loss or gain

- headache or minor illnesses

- rigidity, cynicism, apathy and a general sense of being overwhelmed.

Writing about how we look after ourselves when working with people facing death, dying and bereavement has enabled me to take a fresh look at how I do this for myself. I am certainly aware of how my awareness of the necessity to practise good self-care and obtain regular support and supervision has grown and developed over the years. In reality, we all will find different ways to look after ourselves when doing this work. I hope that my personal experiences will spark ideas for others about their needs and how they might proactively begin to address and meet them. I find it difficult to talk about having a good work/life balance, as we have one life which is made up of many facets and a broad range of different experiences. It is clear to me that when working in end of life care we are constantly confronted by our own mortality as well as the mortality of those we care for and live alongside. The trick is to embrace life and endeavour to sustain an energy which will enable us to enjoy it to its fullest.

Reflection

Attaining and sustaining the right kind and level of support when working in end of life care presents a challenge both for ourselves as individuals and also for the organisations for which we work. What type of appropriate support and supervision structures should be provided for us by the institution and what kind of support do we have the responsibility to seek out for ourselves? What are the downsides of not getting enough support, what issues arise for us when we access and require too much support, and who determines what is enough support and what is too much support anyway?

Being supported and supporting ourselves to do our job of work as effectively as possible should be an imperative for any organisation and professional role. Working with those who are dying or bereaved should be no different. A friend of mine works in the hospitality business and relates to a varied selection of the general public on a daily basis. Some of the experiences she routinely has, and I can only describe them as challenging and complex, are shared with her friends on a regular basis over a glass of wine. She tells us that she also has daily chats with her co-workers, who also share their experiences, and together they support each other to move on and get through the day. However, sometimes she tells us stories which are positive and heart-warming and this, in turn, reminds us that the world also includes people who are good and true. This helps us to realise that, as part of our work, we experience a range of encounters which bring out different responses and reactions in each of us. Maybe something that sustains my friend in her work is the fact that she has an assortment of experiences which range from difficult and complex to joyful and life-affirming, and that she is able to share her experiences from both ends of the spectrum within her different support contexts.

The experiences we encounter on a day to day basis when working in end of life care can indeed be demanding and complicated, but not exclusively so. As with any job, there are high points and low points, achievements to be celebrated and things that go wrong. We know instinctively that sharing the full range of our experiences can be helpful when done as part of both formal and informal processes.

Marion talks about the need to be self-aware, to know ourselves as best as we possibly can. This is where I feel that she gets to the heart of the matter. We are all unique, and as such will require support in different ways. At one time, meeting together with colleagues in a group to discuss something which has affected us will suffice; at another time, speaking through an issue with our manager will help us to unravel a problem; and at another time, sharing something more informally with colleagues or friends will provide the outlet we need in order to move on with our work in a healthy way. Getting to know ourselves and beginning to understand the individual preferences we have for accessing timely and appropriate support is therefore crucial.

It is inevitable that death and dying is frightening. I have worked in end of life care for over 20 years and I am still afraid of what my own death will be like. Working in end of life care does not provide us with a 'buy-out' clause. However, I do realise that when supporting people who are dying, it is not the end of my life and my fear that we are focussing on, and consequently, it is not about me. For myself, I do know that there are a range of support possibilities available, either those offered by the organisation such as support groups and managerial supervision, or sharing and talking with my peers in a more informal way. I also know that shopping makes me happy, that I enjoy a glass of wine or two, and that going to the gym can act as a kind of release which I find enormously helpful.

Taking time to get to know ourselves, to grow our self-awareness and to continue to understand 'this intimate stranger I call me' (Mayne 2002) should be a consistent part of our on-going work and development. Cultivating a more assured self-awareness will enable us to recognise the kind of support mechanisms we prefer to access at different times, and to also recognise the times when we are just expecting too much, either from our patients, our colleagues, ourselves, or indeed from the organisations which we work for.

At the times when I am feeling overwhelmed and when nothing seems to help, I find that it is usually time for a holiday. We must also not underestimate the usefulness of taking a short amount of time out for ourselves in order to put things into perspective.

References

De Hennezel, M. (1999) *Intimate Death – How the Dying Teach us to Live.* London: Vintage Books.

Hartley, N. (2001) 'On a personal note: A music therapist's reflections on working with those who are living with a terminal illness.' *Journal of Palliative Care 17*, 3,135–141.

Lee, C. (1996) *Music at the Edge – The Music Therapy Experiences of a Musician Living with AIDS.* Didcot: Routledge.

Mayne, M. (2002) *Pray, Love, Remember.* London: Darton, Longman & Todd.

Mayne, M. (2002) 'This Intimate Stranger.' Keynote speech given at 10th World Congress of Music Therapy, Oxford.

Monroe, B. (2004) 'When Professionals Weep.' Unpublished Powerpoint Presentation, St Christopher's Hospice.

Renzenbrink, I. (2004) *Living with Dying – A Handbook for Health Practitioners in End of Life Care.* Columbia, NY: Columbia University Press.

Renzenbrink, I. (2011) *Caregiver Stress and Staff Support in Illness, Dying and Bereavement.* Oxford: Oxford University Press.

Thic Nhat Hanh (1991) *Peace is Every Step: The Path of Mindfulness in Everyday Life.* London: Bantam Books.

Weisman, A.D. (1979) *Coping with Cancer.* New York: McGraw Hill Publishing.

Chapter 11

Research and Evaluation

Giorgos Tsiris and Nigel Hartley

Introduction

Research and evaluation have always been part of the trio which makes up the provision of good quality end of life care, the other two parts being the care itself, and the need to influence others through education. However, with regard to the arts and the arts therapies, this is not necessarily the case. Problems with both exploring and comprehending the creative arts lead us to a concept that is increasingly utilised by practitioners across a range of health care settings, but is often neglected by researchers and academics due to its elusive and multifaceted nature. Artists working in health care have also, on the whole, been reluctant to engage in research and evaluation processes, Health care institutions have also been equally reluctant to fund research initiatives into the arts. However, it has become increasingly clear that, in order for the arts to be taken seriously within the changing landscape of health and social care, developing suitable research paradigms which will be able to evidence the efficacy of creative arts work in health care settings has become an imperative. Over the past 20 years or so, there are many examples of artists (Liamputtong and Rumbold 2008; Starikof 2004) and arts therapists (Gilroy and Lee 1995; Ansdell 1995) who have championed research and evaluation as an essential part of their work and successfully investigated the efficacy of the creative arts in a range of different health care settings utilising an expanding range of research and evaluation models and techniques.

In this chapter we meet Giorgos, who is a musician and music therapist at St Christopher's Hospice. Here we witness another example of the importance and potential of offering placements to students as part of their arts or arts therapies training programmes. Giorgos came to St Christopher's as a music therapy student on placement around three years ago, and we were able to offer him paid work following his placement due to the acquisition of some restricted funding. For any arts project we undertake at St Christopher's, the addition of a research, or simple evaluation element is a crucial aspect. Employing arts practitioners who are both interested and capable of fulfilling such a requirement is vital.

Following an introduction where we hear about some of Giorgos's background and motivation for being involved in working in end of life care, and particularly his interest in inquiring into the efficacy of practice, we are presented with some useful information about how to set up simple research and evaluation projects when working as an artist or arts therapist in end of life care. This information is structured in the following way:

- The many facets of evidence gathering

- Basic research steps

- Research ethics considerations

- Developing a collaborative research stance

- Hospices as resourceful organisations

- Looking beyond the organisation

- Two evaluation examples from St Christopher's.

The chapter ends with my reflection.

Giorgos: my background

My name is Giorgos Tsiris, and over the past three years I have been working as a music therapist at St Christopher's Hospice and as a research assistant at the Research Department of Nordoff Robbins, a national music therapy charity (www.nordoff-robbins.org.uk). I first came to St Christopher's as a student when training for the Master of Music Therapy degree at the Nordoff Robbins Music Therapy Centre in London. Prior to this I worked as a special education teacher in my home country of Greece. While on placement at St Christopher's, I learned how broad the work of a music therapist can be and worked with patients in one to one music therapy sessions and also ran a variety of different groups.

From an early stage in my life, I experienced music as something much more than organised sound. I experienced music's power to transform and bring a positive change into people's lives. I could recognise music's potential to affect and connect people irrespective of their age or condition, and in this respect, I recognised that music works. However, this was not enough for me. I was interested to explore and understand *how* music works. I felt the inherent need to understand how one can actually help people through music. This spirit of inquiry, as well as my love for music and people, grew over the years and informed my identity as a reflective practitioner. In 2005, I conducted my undergraduate research in music improvisation and its impact on the interaction skills of people with autism (Tsiris 2005). This was a milestone in my development as a professional, which led me into teaching music to people with special needs and being involved in a number of other projects within the special music education field, such as the development of observation and assessment tools (Tsiris and Kartasidou 2006) and the conduction of a survey exploring special music teachers' perceptions (Kartasidou and Tsiris 2007).

Some years later I trained as a music therapist at the Nordoff Robbins Music Therapy Centre in London where my spirit of inquiry about music's therapeutic power was fostered and grew further to form my current practitioner-researcher identity. Since then my practitioner-researcher identity is constantly informed and shaped by the dynamic interplay between my on-going music therapy practice with dying adults and their families on the one hand, and my research work in the wider field of music, health and wellbeing on the other.

The skills, knowledge and experiences I bring from my music therapy practice and research experience are blended creatively, providing a research insight into practice and a practice insight into research. From this point of view, my research stance and methods are constantly informed by therapeutic work, and vice versa. This blending fosters a critical stance towards the creative tension between the so-called need for evidence-based practice and the vision for practice-based evidence. Many of the ideas presented here have grown not only from my experience at St Christopher's, but also from close collaboration with colleagues at the Nordoff Robbins Music Therapy Centre Research Department, and I would like to acknowledge and express my gratitude to each of them.

My practitioner-researcher identity has a direct impact on my work at St Christopher's where I work alongside my artist colleagues in a range of research-related initiatives. Over the years the team of artists has conducted a number of evaluation projects assessing the impact of its services (some examples are given later on). The conduct of these projects has been guided by a range of restricted funding projects where an objective of the funding has been to evaluate the work and produce a report highlighting the major achievements, and also by St Christopher's wider research culture and infrastructure which has been prominent since the hospice's inception.

The many facets of evidence gathering

It is widely thought that research should be closely interwoven with the development of an organisation's services as well as with its education and training activities. Over the years, St Christopher's has been an exemplar of this. However, I have learned that it is important to keep in mind that a hospice's research programme has many facets and encompasses a range of evidence-gathering processes or pathways. Some of these may fall under what is called research (in the strict sense of the term), but others will be described as audit, evaluation or monitoring. All these are different pathways to evidence-gathering and will serve different aims, have different ethics implications and provide different types of outcomes. Over the years, of course, various discussions regarding what differentiates research from other evidence gathering pathways have also emerged (and faded). Table 11.1 attempts to provide an overview of some of the differences between these pathways.

Table 11.1: Pathways of evidence gathering

	Monitoring	Evaluation	Audit	Research
Aims	To document systems, people or organisations in order to take note of changes over time.	To assess how effective a service is and how it can be improved.	To assess whether a service is following predetermined standards of best practice.	To test and build theory, develop new knowledge, and/or (re-) test research hypotheses.

Function	Documents the service without determination of merit or worth.	Assesses the service as being delivered alongside its aims.	Assesses the service against pre-set benchmarks.	Addresses defined questions, aims and objectives.
Implications	Implications for the service development and its context (site/sector/funder).			Implications for practice, professional knowledge and academic scholarship.
Participants	Anyone directly or less directly affected by the service (e.g., service users, families, staff).			Selected purposively or randomly, depending on project aims, methodology and design.
Intervention	Documenting the standard service being delivered.	Documenting the standard service being delivered and possibly some additional interventions (e.g., interviews, questionnaires).		Studying of existing practice or designing and carrying out interventions in either a laboratory context or in everyday service settings.
Research ethics	Research ethics review not necessarily required, but ethical implications need to be communicated to an ethics representative within the organisation.			Research ethics approval is required.

This table is an adaptation from the book *Towards Ethical Research: A Guide for Music Therapy and Music and Health Practitioners, Researchers and Students*
Source: Farrant, Pavlicevic and Tsiris 2011, p.8

For simplicity, the word 'research' is used as a generic term throughout this section to reflect any type of systematic evidence-gathering pathway (including audit, evaluation, monitoring and research itself). Bruscia's description of research is of relevance here:

> Research is a systematic, self-monitored enquiry which leads to a discovery of new insights which, when documented and disseminated, contributes to or modifies existing knowledge or practice. (Bruscia, cited in Ansdell and Pavlicevic 2001, p.19)

Before embarking on a project, however, practitioners need to have a basic understanding of the differences between the various evidence-gathering pathways, as their differences will impact directly on the implementation and outputs of their project. Comparisons between the different pathways which imply power relationships (e.g., research is 'superior' to evaluation) hold no relevance and can only confuse one's choice. Practitioners are simply encouraged to think carefully which pathway would be appropriate for the aims, needs and context of their own project.

Basic research steps

Generally speaking, each research project will have three main phases: 1. planning, 2. data collection and analysis, and 3. writing up and dissemination of findings.

1. Planning

    Planning includes the selection of an appropriate evidence-gathering pathway, as well as the preparation of a research proposal and any relevant data collection tools, such as questionnaires, interview schedules and so on (Ansdell and Pavlicevic 2001). Planning can be time consuming. However, time is well invested at this phase as this is where the foundations upon which the whole research project is built are set down. By the end of the planning phase, a clear and concise research plan needs to be in place where the following are addressed:

    • *Research aims and questions:* here it is important to distinguish the research aims from the aims of the service (or practice) which is studied or assessed.

- *Research participants and recruitment methods:* research ethics considerations are central here especially when the participants are vulnerable people such as terminally ill or bereaved people.

- *Data collection and analysis methods:* these methods need to be in harmony with the research project aims and questions, as well as the research context. Data collection tools (e.g., questionnaires or interview schedules) have to be sensitive and relevant to participants and their needs (extra care is required when participants are vulnerable people). This does not mean avoiding asking 'difficult' questions, but it requires sensitivity about how and when these questions are asked.

- *Timeline:* the time framework of the project needs to take into account the deadline for the research report delivery, any potential funding deadlines which might be relevant to the project, as well as the amount of time that each researcher can invest on the project. Here, I have discovered that it is important not to underestimate how time consuming simple practical procedures, such as transcribing interview recordings and photocopying, can be.

- *Budgeting:* this includes any potential financial implications including both human resources (e.g., practitioners' case workload and research skills, working hours, attendance of research training) and material resources (e.g., number of photocopies, purchase of data analysis software). I have found that it is important to work with your manager to ensure that this information is as clear as possible.

In all cases, the preparation of a research proposal should meet the specific proposal details required by each organisation. For this reason, I have learned that it is wise to check what the organisation's requirements are at an early stage.

2. Data collection and analysis

In the literature one can find numerous debates and arguments about quantitative versus qualitative research methods. As Daykin writes:

Nevertheless, there is still a debate about what constitutes robust evidence and within the broader arts for health field there is an identified concern that too much emphasis on quantitative outcomes research may inhibit recognition of, or even damage, important arts processes. (Daykin 2007, p.98)

Without delving into this debate or any kind of ideological rigidities, I would simply encourage practitioners to ensure that their methods are in alignment with their project's research aims and questions. For example, different methods (qualitative and/or quantitative) may be appropriate for exploratory, explanatory or descriptive types of research questions (Hedrick 1994). Also, the data collection and analysis methods have to be tailored according to the nature and the resources of each research context, as well as the nature of the practices (or phenomena) which are being studied (e.g., particular arts processes). I often find that this contextual and functional attitude towards the choice of methods makes the debate about quantitative versus qualitative research redundant.

Here it is worth thinking about the possibility of drawing (and combining) data from more than one data source or method; a process known as 'triangulation' (Sale, Lohfeld and Brazil 2002). This process can enhance the validation and trustworthiness of the findings through cross-exploration and verification of the collected data. Of course, any triangulation process will have to be scheduled right from the planning phase.

3. Writing up and dissemination of findings

Writing a concise research report is a standard practice after the completion of the data collection and analysis phase; indeed it is an expectation. When writing the report, I always tend to keep in mind who the audience is. Is the report, for example, addressed to other arts and health practitioners, to funders, or a hospice's senior management team? Based on this, we need to think what our audience already knows, needs or is interested to know. In most cases, however, reports include the following basic sections: background and context, research aims, data analysis or collection methods, findings, conclusions. In addition, providing a summary or executive report of the project findings is good practice, especially when the report is addressed to funders or managers who may have limited time to read a detailed and long report.

Depending on the project's aims and context, practitioners may also use a range of ways and forums to disseminate their research findings. Doing a presentation to your peer group, preparing (poster or oral) conference presentations, publishing a journal article or writing a summary to be uploaded on your organisation's website are some ideas worth considering (Magee 2007).

An essential part of the project writing up and completion is the identification of the meaning that the research findings hold for the organisation's existing services and their future development. Some key questions that we tend to explore at the completion of each research project are:

- How can we use this project's findings to improve our practices?

- What do the findings tell us about:

  o what we do well and what we do less well?

  o what we need to start or stop doing, and what we need to change?

  o what we need to learn and what to teach?

We find that these questions help to recognise problems, strengths and areas for improvement, all of which are vital for the development of good practice.

Research ethics considerations

As indicated in Table 11.1, certain evidence-gathering pathways (such as evaluation) may not require the approval of a research ethics committee, while others may do so. (For practical guidance and tips regarding research ethics application forms, pathways and procedures with particular reference to the fields of music therapy and music and health, see Farrant *et al.* 2011. Also, a helpful account of suggestions for protecting the interests of patients taking part specifically in palliative care research can be found in Speck 2007.) In either situation, however, being aware of the ethical complexities and implications of research is a necessity.

Research ethics are about safeguarding participants' dignity, rights, safety and wellbeing throughout the research process. In the context of palliative care specifically, one has to think carefully about the benefits and risks that people's involvement may entail. Conducting research with vulnerable people who experience serious illnesses and have a limited life expectancy brings a range of ethical (and practical) complexities which are not to be underestimated (Dileo 2005; Farrant *et al.* 2011). We often need to think carefully about the ethical justification of asking terminally ill, and often dependent, patients to participate in studies, especially when it may require extra time and effort on their behalf. Also, I have found that obtaining informed consent for their research participation may be a challenge, as some people's illnesses may prevent them from having the mental capacity to do so. Also, practitioners occasionally come across cases of grateful service users who find it difficult to refuse to participate in a study, although they may really not wish to do so.

Sensitivity to all these complexities and familiarity with the relevant legislation, such as the Mental Capacity Act (2005), are important. Hospices and similar organisations will have policies and procedures which address and alert staff to such issues. In all cases, practitioners need to think carefully how participants' privacy, confidentiality and anonymity will be protected throughout the research process. In relation to this, data protection and storage issues have to be in place. Having an understanding of the organisation's infrastructure helps practitioners to check whether their research complies with the organisational research governance framework, and whether all research managing and reporting lines are in place. This check helps to detect and prevent any potential misconduct, and clarify people's roles within the research team. Having a complaints procedure in place, as well as ensuring transparency of the research design and procedures, are always important. Even if research ethics review is not required in some cases, practitioners are encouraged to discuss with the ethics representative of their organisation and to find out more about the ethical implications of the project.

In St Christopher's case, as artists, we are encouraged to maintain close relationships with key personnel and relevant group meetings who review and provide constructive feedback to the arts and therapeutic research initiatives. We find that such 'critical friends' are extremely helpful for the optimal and ethical conduct of research activities within the organisation.

Developing a collaborative research stance

Funding for palliative care often comes from a range of different sources. It is likely that most hospices will receive some funding from the NHS, but this will only cover part of the services that they offer. Other funding often comes from charitable funds, legacies, trusts and fundraising donations. It is safe to say that any arts or arts therapies projects will be covered by a complex funding mechanism. Much of the work is funded by short-term project-driven work with clear aims and objectives. These aims and objectives will include some form of evaluation process, and this will be a requirement of the funding being granted. Other funding for arts projects might come from specific charitable trusts, and it is important that the objectives of the trust are read and understood prior to applying for support. This situation of recurring short-term funded projects may create a certain degree of insecurity, but as Grande and Ingleton (2008) report, leading charities also recognise the need for research and development programmes.

Having the relevant research funding, skills and resources, however, does not guarantee effective research engagement. What is also required is a spirit of inquiry which would motivate and feed individuals' and organisations' research vision. Although it may sometimes feel like it, research is not a solo performance; it takes a whole community of people and relates to multiple layers of an organisation's life. A spirit of inquiry which promotes a collaborative research stance is therefore recommended as it will entail the sharing of resources and the development of partnerships both within and beyond the immediate organisation.

Hospices as resourceful organisations

Taking a resource-oriented attitude, I have discovered that there is often a wealth of existing human and material resources within organisations. Practitioners' colleagues bring their own life experiences, professional skills, knowledge and professional networks which can complement their own resources and be of help to the delivery of a research project. In addition to these human resources, each organisation has a range of other resources, including: information technology material, policy documents, databases, infrastructures, leaflets and so on (Tsiris 2012).

Thinking of organisations as living networks of people and material, with their own cultures, histories and wisdom I have found to be at the heart of building collaborative communities of inquiry. Some hospices and similar organisations may have a long research and education history; others may not. In either case, however, each hospice has its own ethos which influences (explicitly or implicitly) the ways that it engages with everyday learning, development and new knowledge. To a degree, this organisational ethos shapes arts therapists' and artists' research engagement. However, it can be the case that the opposite is also true.

Practitioners can look for opportunities to join in existing networks or introduce new partnerships (see Heath *et al.* 2010). In St Christopher's, for example, the artists are invited to participate, as with all members of staff, in the hospice's Research and Audit group. Also, over the years artists employed by St Christopher's have undertaken a number of evaluation initiatives (see Gill 2008). Some recent examples are:

- *The journal club:* an informal reading group where artists and arts students on placement share their reflections on journal articles drawing on their own practices and research initiatives.

- *The library:* the artists have created a small, informal library (using some shelves in their office space) where they can share and exchange their own books and articles regarding arts and therapies in palliative and bereavement care. An informal library catalogue and borrowing system has been developed.

- *Continuing professional development reflection meetings:* these informal meetings provide artists with opportunities to share knowledge, experiences and any material from their own continuing professional development (CPD) activities.

- *South London Arts Forum (SLAF):* the hospice established this open forum which aims to bring together artists who work across South London with people facing end of life issues (including bereavement), the elderly and those living with dementia. SLAF provides opportunities for discussion, support, as well as informal education and training.

- *Arts in Palliative Care symposia:* every other year St Christopher's organises a symposium on the role of the arts practices in end of life care. This symposium attracts a number of arts practitioners and researchers from across the world, and provides opportunities for sharing innovative practice and building networks.

These initiatives foster the development of a learning community and therefore enhance St Christopher's research culture (Hartley and Payne 2008). If you are the only artist or arts therapist working within an organisation, it will be important that you link yourself to other professional groups to achieve and experience some of the elements mentioned above. It is likely, for example, that groups of professional staff will meet regularly for some form of journal club, and it will be important to access such groups as part of your own professional development, as well as being accepted and understood as a professional and serious end of life practitioner.

In addition to the above, perhaps the most vital resource for hospices is patients and families who use the services. Patients, their families and friends who access the hospice services are the most insightful teachers who can help practitioners understand how to improve hospice services and care. Reflecting on Dame Cicely Saunders' words, Baines describes St Christopher's research ethos and collaborative stance which calls practitioners to do research *with* patients (instead of *on* them):

> But for all the advances and research in this [the palliative care] field, it is so important that we do not become people who just go round patients with questionnaires and boxes to tick. We need to remember daily the words of Cicely Saunders. 'I have tried to sum up the demands of this work we are planning in the words "Watch with me".' Our most important foundation for St Christopher's is the hope that in watching we should learn not only how to free patients from pain and distress, how to understand them and never let them down, but also how to be silent, how to listen and how just to be there. (Baines 2011, pp.225–226)

Looking beyond the organisation

In addition to engaging with hospices as resourceful organisations, practitioners (and hospices) are also encouraged to look beyond their own organisation. Many hospices will do this as a matter of course, and have strong successful partnerships, for example, with local academic or educational institutions. It is essential that health care organisations engage with their wider professional and disciplinary contexts by exploring the resources, networks and possibilities which are embedded within these contexts (see Figure 11.1).

The strength of the research and education culture in St Christopher's is heavily based on its collaborative attitude both within and beyond its own organisation. The hospice is actively involved in partnerships with various research and funding institutions, such as the Institute of Psychiatry, the Cicely Saunders Institute at King's College and the Arts Council England. Also, St Christopher's has partnerships with arts therapies training institutions and offers students opportunities to undertake their practice placements at the hospice. Student placements provide significant learning opportunities not only to students, but also to the artists and arts therapists who work at the hospice and also to the organisation as a whole. Students bring new ideas and insights which at times may challenge and further the existing knowledge and practices. Similarly, the hospice's liaison with training institutions is a source of inspiration, and future professional and research developments. Such institutions often offer training sessions for placement supervisors, as well as other learning opportunities which help practitioners to keep abreast with on-going developments and current trends in their own disciplinary and professional field as well as offering opportunities for those involved in teaching prospective artists and arts therapists to keep abreast with changes and current challenges happening on the ground.

Furthermore, practitioners are encouraged to liaise with professional and disciplinary peer groups and networks (for some examples, see the 'Resources' section at the end of this chapter).

Peer groups formed by practitioners and researchers from a range of disciplines can bring advantages such as widening one's epistemological and methodological pallet. I have learned that such liaisons can also help develop skills in explaining concepts specific to my own discipline to those unfamiliar with the discipline. This also offers opportunities for collaboration between practitioners and researchers, something which is considered to be 'an important strategy for strengthening the evidence base for arts and health' (Daykin 2007, p.89).

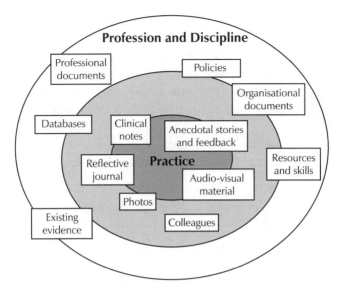

Figure 11.1: Community of inquiry – contexts and resources

Two evaluation examples from St Christopher's

Drawing from the work of artists and arts therapists working at St Christopher's, I now introduce and outline two evidence-gathering projects (which fall under the category of evaluation). These projects were conducted by a range of artists and arts therapists working together and their projects findings were disseminated through poster presentations at international conferences (Hartley *et al.* 2012; Tsiris, Dives and Prince 2010a; Tsiris *et al.* 2012a, 2012b). Based on the original conference poster presentations, the project summaries below aim to give not only ideas about ways of reporting project findings, but also a taste about some research-related initiatives.

Example 1: a music therapy evaluation project

Title: A music therapy evaluation project: Exploring staff's perceptions of music therapy services at St Christopher's

Background: Music therapy is a significant part of the services offered by St Christopher's. It is offered in all contexts of care: The Anniversary Centre (planned day care and outpatients), inpatient wards, home care, care homes and other community venues. Music therapy at the hospice has grown significantly in recent years, offering services through a range of formats (e.g., one to one sessions, groups, community choir, mixed art media projects, concerts, etc.) (Hartley 2008; Tsiris, Dives and Prince 2010b). Music therapists work in collaboration with the wider multi-disciplinary team (MDT) and are involved in the continuing education and training of various professional groups.

Aims: To explore staff perceptions' of the music therapy service at St Christopher's, and identify potential areas for improvement with regards to:

1. the service provision and the music therapists' role and input as part of MDT work;

2. the MDT's understandings of music therapy practice;

3. the effectiveness of the information and communication channels between music therapists and the rest of the MDT members.

Methods: A questionnaire was sent to 168 St Christopher's employees who worked across all hospice contexts. The collected data was numerically and thematically analysed as appropriate. Methodological and ethical aspects of this project were approved by the Research and Audit group, as well as the St Christopher's Research Committee.

Results: The response rate was 48 per cent (80 out of 168). Seventy-one per cent of the MDT members were involved as professionals in nursing and medical care, with 17 per cent in psychosocial and supportive care at the hospice. Eighty-nine per cent had over two years' experience of working at St Christopher's. Fifty-nine per cent were working in the wards, 42 per cent in home care and 24 per cent in the Anniversary Centre (day care and outpatients). The evaluation findings outline five main areas regarding MDT members' perceptions of the music therapy service:

1. *The music therapy service provision*

   Participants' responses highlighted different aspects of the music therapy service which are grouped in the following key themes:

- providing psychological, emotional and spiritual support

- emphasis on therapeutic and professional aspects

- enhancing wellbeing and quality of life

- contributing to management of symptoms

- opportunities for social engagement

- focus on music and music-making.

2. *Common referral reasons to music therapy*

Common MDT members' reasons for referring patients to music therapy are:

- patient's request or personal musical background

- addressing patient's communication and managing aspects of illness

- offering opportunities to patient for emotional expression and psychological support

- enhancing patient's creativity and social participation

- helping patients to express and explore their identity.

3. *Music therapy's impact on patients*

Ninety-five per cent of the participants considered music therapy as being beneficial in general. Five main areas of music therapy's impact on patients were reported: (i) addressing symptoms; (ii) focusing on the patient's healthy aspects; (iii) exploring identity, (iv) enhancing communication and social participation; and (v) addressing psychosocial needs.

4. *Music therapists' input and role in MDT*

Music therapists' role in the MDT was perceived positively by staff, especially with regards to their input in understanding patient's psychosocial conditions and needs, and their contribution to the patients' support plan. Suggestions for improvements included the provision of additional information and in-service staff training with regards to music therapy. Also staff asked for clarification regarding the differentiation between music therapy and the other arts services (i.e., differentiation of goals, processes and roles) in order to help clarify reasons for referral to the different arts modalities.

5. *Communication channels between music therapists and MDT*

Most staff know about music therapy through the music therapists at St Christopher's: informal discussions with the music therapists (64%), music therapists' input in MDT meetings (44%), and music therapists' notes in patients' records (31%). Also, almost half of the participants had heard about music therapy through feedback from other colleagues at St Christopher's (55%), as well as from hospice patients and/or their relatives or friends (47%).

Eighty-five per cent of the participants would like to have more information about the music therapy service. Sixty per cent preferred to be informed through formal presentations or workshops, 50 per cent preferred printed information, and 36 per cent preferred informal discussion with music therapists.

Findings: Staff perceive music therapy as an integral part of St Christopher's MDT work in terms of meeting the holistic needs of dying adults. Further understanding and integration of the music therapy service at the hospice can be encouraged with collaborative work, educational workshops for staff and the development of additional communication channels between music therapists and other MDT members.

Example 2: a community arts evaluation project
Title: An evaluation of the St Christopher's Health Promotion Project

Background and context: The St Christopher's Health Promotion Project is an innovative community arts programme. It takes the form of a short-term collaborative arts project (four weeks) and is part of the hospice's wider community education programme focussing on changing attitudes towards both the work of the hospice and death and dying. The project aims not only to introduce the hospice's work to the public, but also to promote public awareness and change perceptions towards death and dying. It aims to enable relationships to be developed between members of local community groups (such as schools, colleges, pubs and church groups) and patients, families and carers using St Christopher's services (Hartley 2011).

The Health Promotion Project initially involved local schools (St Christopher's Schools Project). Following its success, it has expanded to include the wider community and has recently been rolled out into care homes across South East London (Hartley 2011; Tsiris *et al.* 2011). This Project has been influential at policy level (see DH 2008) and has inspired the development of similar initiatives in various health care organisations both nationally and internationally. To date, St Christopher's has undertaken over 60 projects since 2005. The first systematic evaluation of the Project took place between May and July 2011 (Tsiris *et al.* 2012a, 2012b).

Aims:

- To explore whether and how the St Christopher's Health Promotion Project helps participants to change their attitudes towards death and dying.

- To explore how the arts help people to engage with issues of death and dying, and integrate these concepts into their everyday lives in a healthy and non-threatening way.

Methods: In order to collect perspectives and experiences from different participant groups (e.g., students, hospice patients, artists, etc.) a range of evaluation tools were employed: questionnaires, reflective journals, targeted interviews, attendance at weekly groups' log-sheets, and documentary material. Five projects were targeted reflecting the diversity of communities the hospice works with: four hospice-based projects and one care home-based project. The collected data was analysed both thematically and numerically. The evaluation was approved by the Research and Audit group of St Christopher's.

Summary of results:

- Seventy-eight people took part in this evaluation including hospice patients, students and artists who led the projects.

- The majority of students reported positive changes regarding their attitudes towards art/music, illness, transition and loss in life (see Table 11.2; patients' responses shown in Table 11.3).

- Both students and patients reported that participating in the project was a positive experience for them (students 93%; patients 84%) and they would like to take part in a similar project again (students 95%; patients 92%).

- Three main themes emerge regarding students' changing attitudes:

  1. *Hospices and care homes as non-threatening places:* 95 per cent (n = 56) of the students had not been to a hospice (or a care home respectively) before the project. Despite their initial anxiety and hesitation, students reported positive changes in their attitudes towards hospices or care homes respectively.

  2. *Ageing, illness and death as normal parts of life:* The majority of participants reported a positive change not only in their attitudes, but also in their ways of talking about death and dying with others. This change related also to positive changes in their attitudes towards ageing, illness, as well as towards inter-generational relationships.

  3. *Arts and music as catalysts for change:* Participants' involvement in collaborative art and music-making emerged as a key factor in changing attitudes towards death and dying. Arts and music helped participants to explore meanings with regard to death, dying and transition in life. Also, the arts provided people opportunities for discovering and focussing on each other's resources and abilities.

- People's engagement with the arts was identified as a key area of the project by all participants who reported that their arts engagement engendered a sense of companionship as well as the development of social connections and bonds.

- Both students and patients reported that the project helped them to learn and develop new skills, as well as to become aware of their own resources and resilience in dealing with transition and loss in life.

Table 11.2: Students' reported changes of attitudes

Change of students' attitudes about	Positive change	No change	Negative change
art and music	35	22	0
hospices (or care homes)	52	5	2
very ill people	51	5	2
death and dying	37	16	5
Total responses per category	175	48	9

Table 11.3: Patients' reported changes of attitudes

Change of patients' attitudes about how they	Positive change	No change	Negative change
feel about art and music	5	7	0
feel about their art/music skills	6	3	0
experience illness, transition and loss in life	2	6	1
talk about death and dying?	1	8	0
Total responses per category	14	24	1

Findings and future directions: The St Christopher's Health Promotion Project helps by raising people's awareness of, and promoting healthier attitudes towards, illness, death and dying. The project highlights the central role that the arts can play in the field of palliative and bereavement care, and particularly in health promotion and public death education. The St Christopher's Health Promotion Project is currently expanding into other health care contexts and community groups with the hope of transforming caring cultures by focussing on their ecology, and bringing them in touch with their local communities. The evaluation outcomes inform the development of the St Christopher's death education programme and community work. Also, the outcomes will hopefully benefit other organisations seeking to effectively employ the arts for community engagement in the field of death and dying.

Conclusions: To conclude, I would like to encourage arts therapists and artists, as I have been encouraged, to engage with evidence-gathering procedures by making them an integral part of their thinking and everyday practice. Here, it is important to acknowledge and reassure practitioners that a certain degree of panic is expected when one is about to embark on a journey as a novice researcher. In their book *Beginning Research in the Arts Therapies*, Ansdell and Pavlicevic write:

> Be reassured straight away that a certain amount of panic is only to be expected if you've trained primarily as a practitioner in an arts therapy and suddenly find, for whatever reason, you need to do research...only in recent years have arts therapists become involved in researching their own work (rather than have it researched by professional researchers). Each of the arts therapies now has a number of 'research experts' in their midst, as well as students on Master's level training courses who are learning research methods and producing dissertations. A growing body of home-grown research is resulting from their efforts. (Ansdell and Pavlicevic 2001, pp.9–10)

Today, a decade after the publication of Ansdell and Pavlicevic's book, the research culture, education and body of evidence has grown significantly within the arts and the arts therapies (see also Karkou and Sanderson 2005). Looking into the future, however, one of the biggest challenges perhaps that practitioners (as well as educational and professional bodies) will have to face is the cultivation of a practitioner-research culture, a culture where evidence-based practices are in mutual dialogue with practice-based evidence. This will continue to be tricky in a cash-strapped world, as artists and arts therapists will continue to be employed to work part time. This will mean that providing a service to as many people as possible will understandably and necessarily limit the time needed for consistent in-depth examination and inquiry. Therefore, practitioners will need to explore, discover and utilise both cost and time effective methods of continuing to gain the necessary insights required into the efficacy of the creative arts if they are to continue to be an important aspect of good end of life care.

Reflection

It is clear from Giorgos's account that he holds a palpable interest and passion for inquiry into the work that he does, as well as into the work of his colleagues who he practises alongside. This passion and interest is an important element when it sits within a team of artists, or team of other professionals for that matter, where a number of people from the same professional discipline can share the necessary workload, all with their own specific skills and interests. My experience has shown that it is somewhat more acceptable and possible that one person in the team takes more of their designated work time to focus on the evaluation aspects of the work both they and their colleagues engage in, while others, for example, focus on either clinical work, planning or teaching. However, when you are a lone practitioner, especially working within an organisation part time, this can be particularly problematic and challenging. Giorgos speaks of the cultivation of a practitioner-researcher culture, where practice and research influence each other equally. As a sole arts practitioner employed to work part time within an end of life care organisation, if might be slightly overwhelming to think about how you might set up and provide some kind of comprehensive arts service to patients and families. Add into this the need to educate colleagues and potential referrers about the work that you do, publish and present written information about the service, together with the necessity to evaluate and audit your emerging practice and we begin to see the potential constraints.

I often encounter a gap in expectations when hearing of some people's experiences of either working as, or employing, an artist in end of life care. It is likely that there will be expectations from funders, who will insist on certain outcomes as a prerequisite for investing their funding in a particular arts project. Part of these expectations may be the need for a final written report highlighting the efficacy of the work undertaken with the money provided. From an employer's perspective, the expectations may be different again. They may require a certain number of patients and family members to be worked with during the life of the project, as well as a number of presentations to staff and key stakeholders to be given at key points during the project. The artist or arts therapist might expect to work mostly one to one with patients in a designated room, or to set up a number of 'closed' groups. The artist or arts therapist may also be heavily influenced by any professional bodies to which they belong. Patients and families again, will have another set of expectations, where they might wish to create legacies, arrange funerals, or just to have a good time with arts materials. It is interesting how many times that these expectations do not match up and how the tension created leads to many unfulfilled projects and potential long-term investments in the arts.

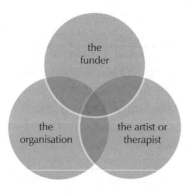

Figure 11.2: Matching up expectations

It is therefore important to match up these expectations from the start, and it may well be the role of the potential artist or arts therapist to take the lead on making this a priority. This will need to be undertaken with a view on what is possible depending on the time available for the work, for example, two or three days a week for a one-year project. In an ideal world, it will be useful to respond to the expectations arising from each area adding practice development alongside evaluation imperatives, mapping in presentations and sessions with patients and families to explain what is possible – all of this while keeping an eye on an effective, concluding report for the funders. After all, it may be this report that helps to secure further funding for future work. However, in my view, the artist or arts therapist will inevitably need to be as flexible as possible when attempting to do this. It is not our role to tell organisations or people what they need and what is best for them, but to listen and to respond, and deliver a service as effectively as possible.

We must remember that research and evaluation is not as frightening or as impossible as it might sound. Personally, I have never been a great researcher into the efficacy of the creative arts, although I have practised and utilised the arts widely over a period of 25 years. However, when I did practise as a music therapist, I was encouraged to follow the discipline of tape recording every music therapy session and then listening back to the recordings of the music created while making detailed notes regarding what I heard. This discipline indeed gave me new insights into the work that I was doing, which in turn influenced how I spoke about what I did, how I wrote about what I did and how I taught other people to do what I did. I am sure that the discipline supported me, not only to develop my personal practice, but also to write successful funding bids and discover a language which continues to convince people of the value of both music therapy and the wider application and efficacy of the creative arts. Giorgos quotes Ken Bruscia as saying that 'Research is a systematic, self-monitored enquiry which leads to a discovery of new insights' (Bruscia, cited in Ansdell and Pavlicevic 2001, p.19). As such, if you have been taught well and take your work seriously, it is likely that you are doing it, in some form, already. The secret might be to simply take time in order to articulate and capture your findings. Reflection on practice is a professional necessity, particularly when working in an acute health care setting. As such, we all have a responsibility and a necessity to live our working lives both as practitioner-researchers and as researcher-practitioners with an attention to detail which safeguards us from the demons of fear and panic.

Resources

This section provides a selected list with research-related web links. Although this list is mainly music therapy and UK focussed, practitioners from other professional or geographical contexts may find it useful.

Research centres and networks

- The British Association of Art Therapists (BAAT) Art Therapy Practice Research Network, www.baat.org/atprn.html

- The British Association for Music Therapy (BAMT) Palliative and Bereavement Care Network, www.bamt.org/british-association-for-music-therapy-mentors/british-association-for-music-therapy-networks/palliative-and-bereavement-care-network.html

- The British Association for Music Therapy (BAMT) Research Network, www.bamt.org/british-association-for-music-therapy-mentors/british-association-for-musictherapy-networks/research-network.html

- Centre for Research into the Arts as Wellbeing, www.winchester. ac.uk/research/attheuniversity/facultyofarts/researchcentres/ artsaswellbeing/Pages/Arts%20As%20Wellbeing.aspx

- The Grieg Academy Music Therapy Research Centre (GAMUT), http://helse.uni.no/Default.aspx?site=4&lg=2

- The International Centre for Arts Psychotherapies Training in Mental Health (ICAPT), Central and North West London NHS Foundation Trust, www.cnwl.nhs.uk/resources/health-professionals/icapt/

- The International Centre for Research in the Arts Therapies (ICRA), (launched in 2009 at Imperial College London and runs in collaboration with the Central and North West London NHS Foundation Trust)

- The Music for Health Research Centre (MHRC), Anglia Ruskin University, www.anglia.ac.uk/ruskin/en/home/microsites/ music_for_health_research_centre.html

- Nordoff Robbins Research Department, www.nordoff-robbins. org.uk/content/what-we-do/research-and-resources

- Sidney de Haan Research Centre for Arts and Health, www. canterbury.ac.uk/Research/Centres/SDHR/Home.aspx

Research ethics and funding

- The Music Therapy Charity, a funding organisation for music therapy research, www.musictherapy.org.uk/mtcstructure.html

- The National Research Ethics Service, www.nres.nhs.uk

Online resources

- The Nordoff Robbins Evidence Bank (2nd Edition, 2012), a collection of music therapy and music and health references and resources, www.nordoff-robbins.org.uk/content/what-we-do/research-and-resources/resources

- Presenting the Evidence (2nd Edition, 2009), the up to date guide for music therapists responding to demands for clinical effectiveness and evidence-based practice, www.nordoff-robbins.org.uk/sites/default/files/Presenting%20The%20Evidence_1.pdf

- The BAMT (British Association for Music Therapy) Register of Surveys, Research and Evaluation Projects (ROSREP), www.bamt.org/display.aspx?iid=2392

References

Ansdell, G. (1995) *Music for Life.* London and Philadelphia, PA: Jessica Kingsley Publishers.

Ansdell, G. and Pavlicevic, M. (2001). *Beginning Research in the Arts Therapies: A Practical Guide.* London: Jessica Kingsley.

Baines, M. (2011). *From pioneer days to implementation: Lessons to be learnt. European Journal of Palliative Care 18,* 5, 223–227. Available at www.stchristophers.org.uk/about/history/pioneeringdays, accessed on 4 October 2012.

Daykin, N. (2007). 'Context, Culture and Risk: Towards an Understanding of the Impact of Music in Health Care Settings.' In J. Edwards (ed.), *Music: Promoting Health and Creating Community in Healthcare Contexts.* Newcastle: Cambridge Scholars Publishing.

Dileo, C. (2005). *Ethical Precautions in Music Therapy Research.* In B. Wheeler (ed.), *Music Therapy Research.* 2nd Edition. Gilsum, NH: Barcelona.

DH (Department of Health) (2008). *End of Life Care Strategy: Promoting High Quality Care for all Adults at the End of Life.* London: DH.

Farrant, C., Pavlicevic, M. and Tsiris, G. (2011). *Towards Ethical Research: A Guide for Music Therapy and Music & Health Practitioners, Researchers and Students.* London: Nordoff Robbins.

Gill, A. (2008). 'Music and Music Therapy at St Christopher's Hospice: An Evaluation Study.' In N. Hartley and M. Payne (eds), *The Creative Arts in Palliative Care.* London: Jessica Kingsley Publishers.

Gilroy, A. and Lee, C. (eds) (1995) *Art and Music Therapy and Research.* London: Routledge.

Grande, G. and Ingleton, C. (2008). 'Research in Palliative Care.' In S. Payne, J. Seymour and C. Ingleton (eds), *Palliative Care Nursing: Principles and Evidence for Practice.* Maidenhead: McGraw-Hill.

Hartley, N. (2008). 'The arts in health and social care – is music therapy fit for purpose?' *British Journal of Music Therapy 22,* 2, 88-96.

Hartley, N. (2011). 'Letting It Out of the Cage: Death Education and Community Involvement.' In S. Conway (ed.), *Governing Death and Loss – Empowerment, Involvement and Participation.* Oxford: Oxford University Press.

Hartley, N. and Payne, M. (2008). *The Creative Arts in Palliative Care.* London and Philadelphia, PA: Jessica Kingsley Publishers.

Hartley, N., Tsiris, G., Lawson, V., Prince, G. *et al.* (2012). 'Why music and arts in death education? Evaluation outcomes from the St Christopher's Health Promotion Project.' Poster presentation at the 19th International Congress on Palliative Care, 9-12 October, Montreal, Canada.

Heath, B., Lings, J., Travasso, R. and Tsiris, G. (2010). 'The Palliative and Bereavement Care Network (PBCN).' *BSMT News, August,* 4-5.

Hedrick, T.E. (1994). 'The quantitative-qualitative debate: Possibilities for integration.' *New Directions for Program Evaluation 61*, 45-52.

Karkou, V. and Sanderson, P. (2005). *Arts Therapies: A Research-Based Map of the Field.* London: Elsevier.

Kartasidou, L. and Tsiris, G. (2007) 'The Lesson of Music for Individuals with Special Needs: A Pilot Study for the Opinions of Music Teachers in Greece.' In P. Simeonides, P. Androutsos, D. Paklatzi and D. Koniari (eds) *Proceedings of the 5th Conference of the Greek Society for Music Education, 'Music Education and Search of Cultural Identity'* (pp.160–168). Thessaloniki: GSME.

Liamputtong, P. and Rumbold, J. (eds) (2008) *Knowing Differently: Arts-based and Collaborative Research Methods.* New York: Nova Science Press.

Magee, W. (2007). 'Focusing on Outcomes: Undertaking the Music Therapy Research Journey in Medical Settings.' In J. Edwards (ed.), *Music: Promoting Health and Creating Community in Healthcare Contexts.* Newcastle: Cambridge Scholars Publishing.

Pavlicevic, M., Ansdell, G., Procter, S. and Hickey, S. (2009). *Presenting the Evidence: The up to date Guide for Music Therapists Responding to the Demands for Clinical Effectiveness and Evidence-Based Practice.* London: Nordoff Robbins.

Sale, J.E., Lohfeld, L.H. and Brazil, K. (2002). 'Revisiting the quantitative-qualitative debate: Implications for mixed-methods research.' *Quality & Quantity 36*, 1, 43-53.

Speck, P. (2007). 'How to Gain Research Ethics Approval?' In J. Addington-Hall, E., Bruera, E., Higginson, I. and Payne, S. (eds), *Research Methods in Palliative Care.* Oxford: Oxford University Press.

Starikof, R. (2004) *Arts in Health: A Review of the Medical Literature.* Research Report 36. London: Arts Council England.

Tsiris, G. (2005) 'The use of musical improvisation to enhance the interaction of individuals with autism: A case study.' Unpublished undergraduate thesis. Department of Special Education, University of Thessaly.

Tsiris, G. (2012). 'Responding to the needs for evidence.' Invited presentation at the Annual Conference of Key Changes Music Therapy, 28 April, Winchester University.

Tsiris, G., Dives, T. and Prince, G. (2010a). 'A music therapy evaluation project: Exploring staff's perceptions of music therapy services at St Christopher's.' Poster presentation at the 'First National Symposium for the Arts and Creativity in End of Life Care', 5-6 November, St Christopher's Hospice, London.

Tsiris, G., Dives, T. and Prince, G. (2010b). 'Music therapy at St Christopher's hospice.' *BSMT News, August,* 13-15.

Tsiris, G. and Kartasidou, L. (2006) 'Parameters of Planning and Implementation of Music Educational-therapeutic Programs in Special Education.' In I. Etmektsoglou and C. Adamopoulou (eds) *Music Therapy and the Music Approaches for Handicapped Children and Adolescents* (p.153). Athens: Nikolaidis.

Tsiris, G., Tasker, M., Lawson, V., Prince, G. *et al.* (2011). 'Music and arts in health promotion and death education: The St Christopher's Schools Project.' *Music and Arts in Action 3,* 2, 95-119. Available at http://musicandartsinaction.net/index.php/maia/article/view/stchristophersschoolsproject/57.

Tsiris, G., Tasker, M., Lawson, V., Prince, G. *et al.* (2012a). 'Music, arts and death education: The St Christopher's Health Promotion Project.' Poster presentation at the 9th Palliative Care Congress, 14-16 March, Newcastle.

Tsiris, G., Tasker, M., Lawson, V., Prince, G., Dives, T. and Sands, M. (2012b). 'Music, arts and death education: The St Christopher's Health Promotion Project.' *British Medical Journal Supportive and Palliative Care 2:* A113. Available at http://spcare.bmj.com/content/2/suppl_1/A113.1.abstract.

Chapter 12

Final Thoughts and Some Handy Hints and Tips

Final thoughts

In this concluding chapter, I set out some of the key arguments for the inclusion of the arts, therapies and arts therapies professions within the health and social care framework, highlight some of the key issues raised throughout, and also incorporate 'Ten Handy Hints and Tips' for the professional who wishes to work within this particular arena.

I began by highlighting the importance of understanding strategy and the organisational 'story' in order to successfully place both practitioner and profession within the end of life care workplace.

Below we are reminded of how the current economic and humanitarian crisis affects ourselves as practitioners, those we provide care to, the organisations we work for and the world at large:

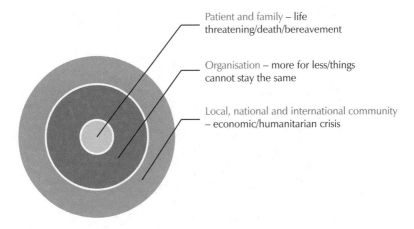

Figure 12.1: Different levels affected in a crisis

Creativity

It is important at the time that this book is being written for us all to ask ourselves some important questions:

- How can we be the best we can be and do the best job that we can?

- What does this look like when it is achieved from a whole professional group and organisational perspective?

- How can we, through our work, support groups and communities of people to work together to be the best they can be?

We can see examples of the benefits of striving to be the best we can be and working as effectively as possible together for the good of others throughout this book. The need for creative individuals has never been greater. It is widely known that creative individuals can support creative organisations, which can in turn lead to creative communities (Kotter 1996).

We only need to examine the life and work of some of the great artists and creative practitioners to witness the benefits to bring both to organisations and to society in general (Csikszentmihalyi 1996). Some of these include:

- courage

- persistence

- curiosity

- the ability to take risks and to make mistakes

- the ability to discover patterns and to make connections.

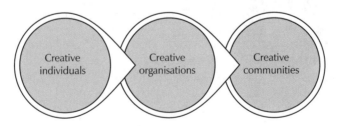

Figure 12.2: Creative individuals

It seems clear, therefore, that health and social care organisations providing services within the current climate can benefit from attracting creative people to support their work and to enable them to be the best they can be. We also experience and witness many times when reading this book that creative people can, as well as provide innovation and motivation, often be responsible for certain challenges for organisations, and experience shows that in some circumstances creativity might need to be harnessed and moulded. This is because some creative ideas and innovations will require translation by organisations into services that funders will pay for and that patients and users want and need, thus balancing new possibilities with demands and expectations. However, new ideas will also need to be fostered within an organisational structure which is not obsessed with bureaucracy and formal controls and is able to think 'beyond risk'. This is not an easy ask, but history does show that we need to trust and have the courage to do something new and different when something new and different is needed. A certain level of confidence and maturity will be required if we are able to live with the fact that from time to time things will go wrong and not let ourselves allow this fact to prevent us from still being able to test and learn new and different ways of doing things.

Reconceptualising dying

It is a major challenge for end of life care to reconceptualise what it is to be dying (Calanzani, Higginson and Gomes 2013). For many, dying happens over a number of years, and we will need to find ways of creatively supporting people through the process over longer periods of time. Therefore, it seems likely that the kind of resources needed to support people more long term will be different than those resources needed for short bursts of care over the last few days of life. Complex pain and symptom management and good, practical nursing will always be vital to enable people to die without distress and in comfort. This will also be important for families and carers whose experience of their family member or friends' death will live with them for the rest of their lives and affect their perceptions of death into the future. However, intense medical and nursing care will not be needed consistently for people living with dying over a period of years rather than months, weeks or days. It is more likely that these people will benefit from more on-going social, creative and therapeutic services and activities for them to be able to begin to make sense of their illness both individually and as part of the communities within which they live and within which they will die.

Why artists, therapists and arts therapists?

It is our hope that the best of what artists, therapists and arts therapists can bring to end of life care rings clear throughout this book. Although the arts and other therapies are not a new addition to end of life care, it is clear that they have often been marginalised and misunderstood (Hartley and Payne 2008). Here we remind ourselves of how artists, therapists and arts therapists can positively place themselves as a response to the demands and expectations of both users and end of life care organisations.

Matching up these three areas above is imperative to success:

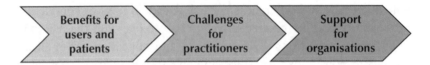

Figure 12.3: The value of mutuality

1. Benefits for users and patients

    We have known for some time that vulnerable people benefit from having access to a variety of opportunities and that one size does not fit all. Much of what we witness throughout this book reminds us that vulnerable people at the end of life, who also include family members, carers, those who are bereaved and communities which are afraid of death and dying, need access to services which can:

    • support them to articulate themselves both to themselves and to others

    • enable them to know that they do still matter

    • bring them together with others outside of sometimes suffocating and controlling networks of families and friends

- challenge the experience of 'social death' which can accompany a terminal diagnosis

- engage with others outside of the 'numbness' of illness and symptoms

- develop and sustain confident and compassionate communities

- enable them to create products and legacy and support 'remembering'

- give people the opportunity to surprise themselves and to develop empowerment and self-efficacy

- help to redress the balance of taking and giving

- offer people a variety of frameworks and contexts in order to understand difficult things and to confront difficult things

- enable people to create order out of chaos

- support people to put relationships right – to discover ways of saying 'I'm sorry' or 'I love you' and so forth.

2. Challenges for practitioners

Throughout many of the chapters, we also see clearly some of the ways of addressing the challenges and questions for arts and therapy practitioners working within the end of life care arena. These include:

- How do we discover more robust ways of articulating success?

- How do we demystify the work that is done and what is achieved?

- How do we move beyond the 'secrecy' of therapy and make the work that we do more visible within the workplace?

- How do we make ourselves indispensable?

- How do we want to be labelled for the future and does it matter?

- How do we know if we are having the 'right debate'?

This final question is an interesting one. It seems important that we should not waste any time talking and arguing from within our professions about issues which are irrelevant and barely matter in the wider scheme of things. In order that we can reassure ourselves that we are on track and also that we are having a useful debate, a dialogue must be kept open between all stakeholders including training institutions, professional bodies, organisations who provide services and those who utilise those services. We must deftly find new ways of understanding each other, working together and articulating what we do, and on this survival and growth depends.

3. Support for organisations

We also note throughout many of the chapters that the arts and other therapies can support organisations successfully in the following ways:

- meeting some strategic imperatives effectively

- providing an impact which outweighs the cost

- attracting responses and reactions

- providing creative and flexible approaches to problems

- impacting on the environment and the everyday life of the organisation

- providing new and different ways of viewing the world

- offering continuously fresh experiences and expanding potential and possibility.

Ten top handy hints and tips

The following handy hints and tips are picked out from the main body of the text of this book where you will have witnessed and experienced some very real and active ways of responding to them. They are intended as an aide memoire in order to support arts and therapy practitioners to stay focussed and engaged in the most useful ways possible.

1. Understand both the strengths and weaknesses of your professional discipline

This will support you to 'place' your profession in the most useful way. What can you realistically help with? How can you make the biggest difference and impact? Which gaps can you fill?

2. Know the environment and the organisation

Researching the area of work you wish to work in will pay dividends. You should also remember that even when working within an end of life care organisation, new information will continue to become available. Persist on searching out new papers, studies and reports which will give you clear information about current and future pressures and potential changes. What information is available? What are the main texts that will be useful to read? Where can you access the most up-to-date information?

3. Be prepared to be flexible

Nothing should be non-negotiable as part of your work. How can you benefit as many people as possible? What are the different contexts within which you are expected to work? Which new organisational ideas can you respond to?

4. Be ready to negotiate on cost

What you charge for your services might inhibit possibilities and it could be useful to lower your cost in order to gain employment. This may be considered contentious, but is worth bearing in mind. Can you agree any incentives with the organisation regarding payment? Is it possible to volunteer some time in order to prove the efficacy of what you offer? Is it possible to find funding for yourself in order to approach a possible employer?

5. Understand your own relationship with death

Although this might appear obvious, it is important not to make an assumption that you can easily deal with death and dying. How can you think about this in advance? How have you responded when people close to you have died? What are your plans/fears for your own death?

6. Explore audit, research and evaluation models and tools

It will be important that you have some ideas to prove that your practice and discipline actually works. What research and evaluation have been done in this area before? How can you offer to include this as part of any work you might be doing? Does the organisation have an on-going research and audit plan, and how might you fit into this?

7. Offer to work in partnership with others

It will be probable that many other professionals and professional groups will be useful allies to work alongside. Potential partners may sit both within and outside of the organisation. Which professional groups might you ally yourself alongside? Which organisations within the community might be useful partnerships both for yourself and your work and also the institution that you are working with? Which partnerships are you able to bring with you which might benefit the organisation?

8. Find a clear way of articulating what you do

This should be a life time's work for any arts or therapies professional working in health or social care. You will need to be able to talk about what you do in a variety of ways to a variety of people. Hopefully this will also help you to understand the uniqueness of what you do and the differences you can bring to the experiences of people both living with dying. Where does the language originate from that you utilise to talk about what you do? Does this language make sense in any or every situation? Can you explain clearly what you do to users, funders, managers and colleagues?

9. Be aware of funding mechanisms

It is likely that any work you are involved in might be supported from a range of complex funding mechanisms. It is important to understand these, as you do not want to waste energy arguing for funding from statutory bodies, when in reality this will be an unlikely source. It also could be foolish to assume that funding for your work will be on-going. Do you know where the money comes from to pay you for the job that you do? How can you make yourself aware of any potential funding possibilities? Are you aware of how to write a funding proposal?

10. Have some fun!

It is generally assumed that consistently working with death and dying can be intense, sad and sometimes depressing. Do not underestimate the importance of laughter and humour both for users of services and those who provide them. How do you relate to the people you work with? Do you include a healthy balance of experiences and opportunities within your work? Are you able to laugh at yourself and with others as part of your work?

Conclusion

We know that there are a number of ways to successfully support vulnerable people who are coming to the end of their lives, as well as to support those who are caring for them. It is true that sometimes the pain and distress that such people experience is too deep to either understand or to even share with others. Therefore, much of the time for professional practitioners there is the potential to be left feeling deskilled, useless, unwanted and unneeded.

However, although we cannot know what it is like to be dying, but there are many common human experiences which we share and which can enable us to sit alongside others who are needing to find the resilience to manage what might seem unmanageable, to bear what appears to be unbearable, or to think about things which, to many of us, might be unthinkable. As human beings we know what it is like to be vulnerable and afraid, to feel alone and anxious as well as to feel joyful, needed and loved. All of these mutual experiences provide us as care givers with platforms where we can be usefully and helpfully together with others in quite ordinary and commonplace ways. If the development of end of life care has been about anything, it has been about letting us know, that in most circumstances, dying is normal and can be managed well. It would be false to say that working in this arena is never difficult or problematic. However, we must also realise that it is no more difficult or complex than any other role or profession.

If this book is about anything, it is about helping and supporting artists, therapists and arts therapists to realise the need to be flexible and up for conversation, the need to get better at articulating what we do, the need to utilise everything we have and all that we are to support vulnerable people faced with death, and the need to continue to be creative and challenging. The test is to do this whilst matching our own agendas with those of the people who can benefit from what we offer, namely users of services, organisations, policy makers and funders, as well as our communities at large.

Dr Robert Twycross ended a eulogy to Dame Cicely Saunders at Westminster Abbey, London in 2006 with the following:

> Palliative care services, even in Britain, generally have not yet reached their full holistic potential. But movements tend to become monuments. So the best tribute that we can give…is to make sure that hospice, that palliative care, remains a movement with momentum. (Twycross 2006)

We hope that everything that has been shared in this book inspires and motivates you to join us as part of this commitment to the future of end of life care services across the world, and to acknowledge the relevant and important part that artists, therapists and arts therapists might play within its on-going development.

References

Calanzani, N., Higginson, I.J. and Gomes, B. (2013) 'Current and future needs for hospice care: an evidence-based report.' *Commission into the Future of Hospice Care.* London: Help the Hospices.

Csikszentmihalyi, M. (1996) 'Implications of a Systems Perspective for the Study of Creativity.' In R.J. Sternbery (ed.) *Handbook of Creativity* (pp.313–336) London: Sage Publications.

Hartley, N. and Payne, M. (2008) *The Creative Arts in Palliative Care.* London and Philadelphia, PA: Jessica Kingsley Publishers.

Kotter, J.P. (1996) *Leading Change.* Boston, MA: Harvard Business School Press.

Twycross, R. (2006) *Eulogy at Dame Cicely Saunders' Memorial Service.* London: Westminster Abbey. Available at www.stchristophers.org.uk.

Contributors

Tamsin Dives trained as a singer at the Guildhall School of Music in 1982 and for 22 years followed a career as an opera and concert singer. In 2005 she returned to train as a music therapist and since qualifying has worked with a range of client groups. She now works at St Christopher's as a music therapist and as a member of the arts team.

Nigel Hartley currently holds the post of Director of Supportive Care, a senior management position at St Christopher's Hospice, London. He has worked in end of life care for almost 25 years more recently working on the redevelopment of day and outpatient services at St Christopher's Hospice before taking on his current position. He has held posts both at London Lighthouse, a centre for those living with HIV/AIDS, and Sir Michael Sobell House, which is a large hospice in Oxford. Nigel was the only person to simultaneously chair the Association of Professional Music Therapists (APMT) and the British Society of Music Therapy (BSMT) which in turn led to the merger of both organisations. He has a postgraduate qualification in management from Ashridge Business School, England. Nigel has an international reputation both as a teacher and a writer in end of life care, focussing on the arts, day care, volunteers, health promotion and social care. He is a trustee of the London Arts in Health Forum (LAHF).

Gini Lawson is an integrative arts psychotherapist, community artist and visual artist. She is a member of the Health Professions Council, the UK Council for Psychotherapy and the British Association of Art Therapists and a member of the special interest group, Creative Response. She works at St Christopher's Hospice and has a private practice working with individuals and groups.

Gerry Prince is a music therapist, session musician and songwriter. Since qualifying as a music therapist, he has worked in a palliative care setting for both St Christopher's and St Joseph's Hospices providing one to one, group and community work as well as student supervision.

Andy Ridley qualified as an art psychotherapist at Goldsmiths College in 2011 and currently works as an art therapist at St Christopher's Hospice and a nursing assistant in oncology at St Bartholomew's Hospital in London. He is a practising visual artist.

Roberto Marcelo Sánchez-Camus is an artistic director and project manager producing works in theatre, circus, visual arts, social interventions and live art. He has devised, directed and managed shows across four continents. His interests focus on participation, community, urbanism and psychogeography. He co-manages Lotos Collective, an immersive theatre company (www.camusliveart.net).

Mick Sands is an artist, musician and theatre composer who regularly performs and records. As well as being a member of the St Christopher's arts team he has a dramatherapy and music therapy practice with adults with learning disabilities.

Marion Tasker trained at Ravensbourne College of Art and Design studying technical and botanical illustration. She worked in audiovisual design and then as an illustrator in medical publishing. As a freelance practitioner her clients include Elsevier, Taylor and Francis, Butterworth Heinemann, HarperCollins and Designers Collective. She is currently completing a degree in counselling at the Metanoia Institute.

Giorgos Tsiris works as a music therapist at St Christopher's Hospice and as a research assistant at Nordoff Robbins. He is the editor-in-chief of *Approaches: Music Therapy and Special Music Education*. He serves as the coordinator of the Research Network of the British Association for Music Therapy. He is conducting his doctoral research on music therapy and spirituality at Nordoff Robbins (City University, London).

Subject Index

Author Index